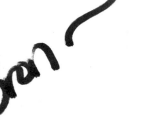

To LeBron~

The
Miracle
Healer

I met in California

You Rock...!!

Pamelarocks

BY

PAMELAROCKS

Cover Image by dreamstime.com

Inside book images by www.dreamstime.com and www.depositphotos.com

Book Cover Design by Pamelarocks

Editor: Linda Gerlt   E-mail address: lindagerlt@yahoo.com

Printed in the United States of America

ISBN #- 978-1981370344

Contact information: miraclehealerincalifornia@gmail.com

Website: www.miraclehealerincalifornia.com

This magical book is
especially created for
those individuals who are suffering
and who may need a
Miracle Healer
to mend their hearts, physical bodies,
and souls.

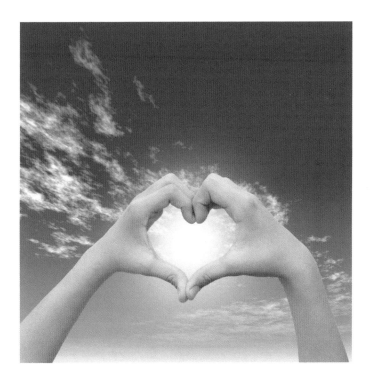

Table of Contents

"When you focus on your own internal world and channel your energy effectively… a human being is limitless in one's own potential."

Master Hai

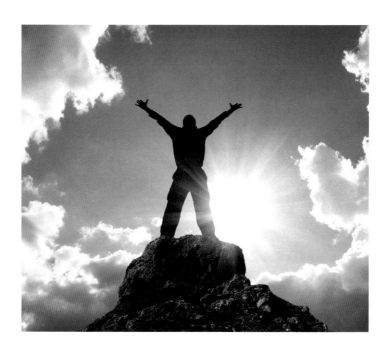

Introduction

Miracle is defined in the 2018 online Merriam-Webster dictionary as:

1) an extraordinary event manifesting as divine intervention in human affairs
2) an extremely outstanding or unusual event, thing, or accomplishment
3) a supremely, awesomely, divinely natural phenomenon experienced humanly as the fulfillment of spiritual law

Have you ever longed for a true miracle in your life? Do you wonder how other people's energy affects you? Do you feel good most of the time or are you suffering with an ailment that affects all areas of your life?

I met a modern-day Miracle Healer. His name is Master Hai. He performs miracles every day by healing the many patients who feel so deeply blessed to have been led to him.

They could only be defined as "Miracles" because they defy explanation or scientific reason. He demonstrates the Power of the Mind with each person he miraculously heals. He is the greatest spiritual power I have ever met on the planet.

I am writing this book for you. I want to share with you the many miracles I witnessed and experienced with a true Miracle Healer I met in California.

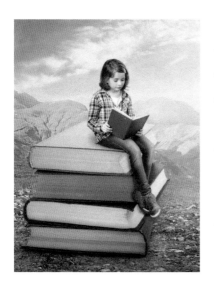

I read about 50 books to prepare to write this book that ranged from great Western medicine textbooks to advanced Chinese medicine textbooks. I immersed myself in the mind-expanding Eastern philosophies.

I also interviewed many health clinics that offer pain relief alternatives such as, but not limited to: physical therapists, chiropractors, and acupuncturists.

I initially thought I was going to try and explain to you, the reader, how Master Hai performs these miracles. My preparation was mind-boggling to me because I could not find one book in any library or at any major bookstore that came close to explaining what he does. Most, if not all of the acupuncture clinics I interviewed were the same, in that they stated they assist the body in healing itself, but did not heal the body.

I discovered many Western medicine books that were written for the average individual to read that included the basics of health, diet, and nutrition.

I found many Eastern medicine and philosophical books that were fascinating

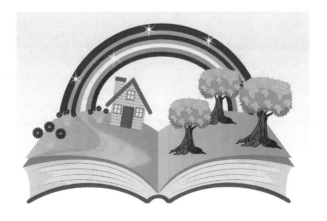

learning experiences for me to read. I was fascinated by the large variety of Buddhist books whose authors described and explained the coveted enlightened state of being. Their goal was to attract and cultivate a sense of grateful mindfulness into all their moments.

I also educated myself by reading books on the topics of acupuncture, body's chakras, and Eastern medicinal ways to heal the body.

However, after weeks of searching for content and researching book material to assist me in writing this book, I could not find one book to explain to you HOW Master Hai heals patients all day long. I realized I had to just tell you my truth.

I do not have any scientific explanations to interject into these carefully written sentences I am creating for you. I only have true testimony from grateful patients who have been healed by Master Hai. I am a witness to his miracles and his patient's success stories are the solid proof detailing his great God-given healing powers.

Master Hai is the greatest, most powerful spiritual being I ever have encountered on this planet. This is my humble attempt to radiate Master Hai's miraculous abilities to you through words, feelings, experiences, and moments.

Get comfortable, get a cup of tea, and enjoy the ride!

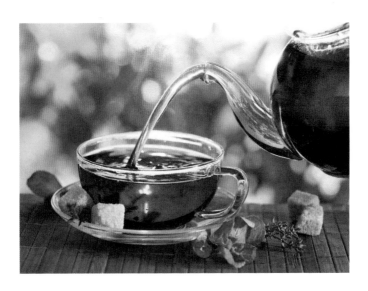

*"I
don't heal,
God heals…
through
me."*

Master Hai

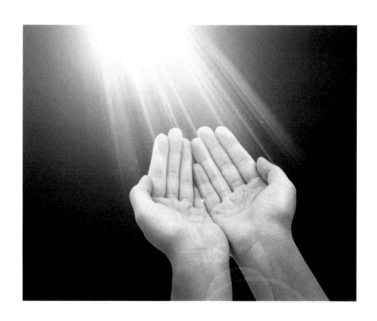

The Doorway to Divine Healing

Most of Master Hai's patients have the same story. They were miraculously guided to Master Hai's doorway after completely running out of options or hope for the ailment or malady they were suffering. They met Master Hai and he healed them.

Master Hai has God-given miraculous gifts that assist him to heal human beings with all types of ailments and sufferings. He does not utilize any tools, equipment, or props. He utilizes his hands and a great inner power, that is like a high-voltage energy, which comes from within his being. The best way to describe his energy is like an electric lightning bolt. Master Hai says the energy he utilizes is the universe's energy, which is always available and replenishes instantly.

Others always ask him how he does this and if he can teach us, however, he says that if we are meant to heal then the gift will be given.

I recall telling him many years ago that I wanted to be able to do what he does and he calmly replied, "You can try." The way he said it was so humorous because I am sure all his patients have said the same thing. Who wouldn't want to learn how to heal themselves and others? All I know is that if he can do it, then it exists on this planet. I may not be able to explain it in scientific terms with graphs or charts, but explaining the unexplainable is my job right now as I write this book for you.

Where does this healing energy come from? The Universe, or God.

I had the honor of witnessing Master Hai perform healing miracles on patients of all ages, sizes, and ethnicities. He invited me to observe him perform these unexplainable miracles in his office for the past year. I have seen Master Hai heal many people with fourth stage cancer, kidney failure, seizures, strokes, emotional or spiritual issues, just to name a few miracles.

I discovered a common denominator with most of Master Hai's patients. They said he was their last hope after knocking on many doors for help and they were about to give up. Once they found Master Hai's doorstep, he became the Greatest Blessing of their lifetime.

I asked Master Hai if I could talk to some of his patients and ask what their experiences were and he allowed me this honor. The patients eagerly told me how they were led to him, what he did and how he healed them, and how they are doing now.

There is no limitation or boundary in regard to what Master Hai can heal. Each patient is unique with individual descriptions of pain, ailments, or suffering. Master Hai simply sees all issues in terms of "removing blocks" or negative energy stagnant in the patient's body.

Master Hai says that it is not himself healing the patients, but that it is God working through him and healing the patients.

The best way to describe the healing energy that Master Hai energetically transmits from his human vessel to the recipient is like an energy current of vibrant life force.

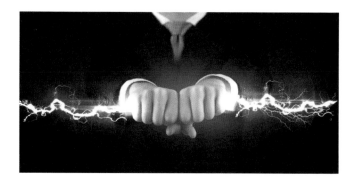

The electric current flows through him like a conduit and he pushes out the stagnant, negative energy that is trapped in the body that was causing or creating the painful symptoms.

Sometimes a person needs more than one treatment to ignite the body's own natural healing processes for optimal results. The body's natural patterns are complex and each person is different and has different reactions to the high-voltage treatments. Multiple treatments for more serious ailments are recommended, however single treatments are often sufficient for less severe cases. Everyone has different results based on their circumstances and he often can tell you immediately what it will take and what he recommends, in terms of how many treatments and length of time to heal.

The results of Master Hai's treatments are outstanding, with noticeable improvements in a short amount of time. Many of his patients eagerly return to Master Hai for tune-ups that are more preventative in nature.

The powerful Qi (chee) life-giving energy that Master Hai transmits to his patients assists the body to heal on all levels. The Qi energy feels like a heating furnace of pure love. It increases your awareness of your life's current created states of being. Your inner world becomes stronger and you begin to desire less of the "outside" world's fleeting distractions.

Master Hai is extremely gifted and channels good energy to his patients, which was the most amazing demonstration of the human mind that I have yet experienced. He says that if we discipline our minds and bodies, that our potential can be limitless.

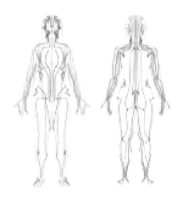

The Body Meridians

Some of the ailments which I have witnessed Master Hai successfully treated are the following, but not limited to: cancers of all types, multiple sclerosis, mental and emotional disorders, strokes, Bell's Palsy, depression, anxiety, concussions, jaundice, TBI, bronchitis and lung failure, seizures, stomach disorders, OCD, acid reflux, IBS, thyroid disorders, digestion problems, acne, skin cancer, kidney problems, bladder infections, common flu/cold, swollen feet, athletic injuries, hair loss, knee and joint ailments, prevented heart attacks, hiccups, gallbladder issues, asthma, TMJ, carpal tunnel syndrome, migraine headaches, thyroid problems, skin rashes, sciatica, whiplash, anemia, hypertension, stress issues, arthritis, circulation problems, ulcers, spine and back issues, food allergies, food poisoning, pancreas issues, diabetes, broken bones, imbalances, spiritual dilemmas, and many more.

The individual's labeling of the ailment is of no concern to Master Hai because he sees ailments mainly in terms of "blockages" in the body's system. Once he infuses the patient with the vital rejuvenating Qi energy, their body begins to heal and push out all the toxins.

The treatments are remarkable and the best way I can explain it to you would be "miraculous"! Many patients expressed to me they feel younger, look younger, and have increased energy and stamina. Master Hai's treatments will flow vibrant new energy into your meridians and channels.

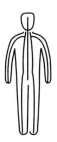

Meridians, or channels, are pathways of our life force that travel throughout the body. They are like the super highways of our body's delicate systems. They are energetic channels that carry oxygen, blood, and necessary flowing nutrients to all areas of our body.

When your body has a blockage in the

flow of a meridian channel, you may experience discomfort and pain. Energy blocks are like traffic jams in your body.

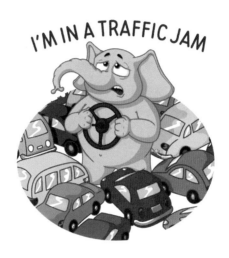

Meridian blocks, or traffic jams, hold up the flow and cause imbalances in your body's system. You may feel a ping, then a pang. You ask yourself what could that be? It's a block. A block is occurring within your system when you feel pain. Flowing energy feels GOOD. Stagnant negative energy feels not so good. Everyone's body must perform so many tasks and duties throughout the day. Often a person is not even consciously aware of all the magical tasks the body performs because it's automatic. Many different systems are working together all at one time. If a part of your body's factory shuts down, it affects your body's ability to perform tasks and you experience a warning sign of discomfort or pain.

Master Hai clears up the traffic jams in your body so everything flows smoothly again!

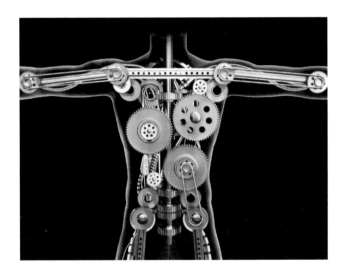

Your body is like a factory with cogs and wheels that must run properly and optimally for best results. The ping-pang sensation is telling you something is not quite right. Some people ignore the pain, or worse, cover it up with medication. Pain is there for a reason. It is the body's way of telling us that it needs help or wants our attention to do something. Pain can be motivating because you have to find a way to relieve it or often it gets worse or causes more problems. Correcting an issue before it gets out of control is always best, however, often we are so busy or distracted that we don't listen, do we?

Master Hai's high-voltage miraculous energy treatments are filled with life-giving Qi (pronounced chee). Qi is considered the vital life force that flows through the body in many Asian cultures and Eastern medicine. Qi is the living and vibrant force that makes us feel GOOD. Master Hai's Qi energy will remove any dormant or negative energy stuck in the body that may be blocking the flow of your vital Qi energy.

Acupuncturists or massage therapists, and other holistic practitioners all have the same goal of repairing or rejuvenating meridian blocks, however, finding a reputable and effective one is often a challenge. Individuals who work with opening up another person's meridian system must be keenly aware of the sensitive nature of such a t ask, as the transferring of energy from the practitioner to the patient is conveyed in that process. Master

Hai is authentic and has been healing patients on a daily basis for over 30 years.

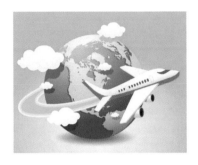

Patients travel in from all over the world to see Master Hai for healing treatments.

He often schedules months out in advance. He never has any cancellations because when you know it's your turn to be healed by his gifts you don't want to miss the appointment, which is such a blessing.

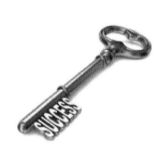

Master Hai says not everyone will be able to find his doorway, because not everyone will find the key. My hope in writing this book is that I put the key in your hand and you will find him.

*"You are fortunate to be so blessed
with the many things you have.*

*Think of what you have,
not what you don't have."*

Master Hai

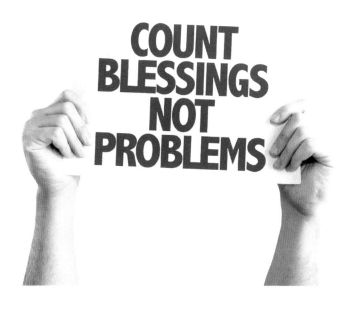

The Treatments

I met a genuine modern-day Miracle Healer named Master Hai in California. He has influenced and changed my fate and my life's path in such a positive way that I am eternally grateful. His amazing treatments are life giving, miraculous and powerful. He is pure, positive energy and wisdom and seeks neither notoriety nor fame. He only wants to heal and help the suffering. He finds joy in each day that he can change someone's life in a positive, miraculous way.

Eastern medicine's form of acupuncture or acupressure would be the closest term to associate or describe what he is doing, with the added benefit of the high-voltage energy he transmits to the patient called Qi (life force). He doesn't use needles or equipment, just his hands and his life force.

In my opinion, his fees are affordable so that anyone can come see him who needs him. I personally feel that his treatments are worth about a million dollars a session!! I say that because the positive effects of the treatments extend far beyond just healing the illness that brought the patient to him. They enhance a person's entire being that includes the emotional, mental, and spiritual world.   His healing energy raises the vibration of the patient with the domino effect of enhancing their family, partners, workplace, community and friends.

Treatments are scheduled weeks, or months out, because the line of people is quite long to get a chance to see Master Hai. I have waited months sometimes for a scheduled treatment. When the day arrived, I was so excited because of the consistent and positive results of the treatments. I appreciated the opportunity to see him again.

Master Hai increases and raises a person's Qi (life force) energy levels so the body can heal itself naturally.   Qi is the life force energy that ebbs and flows throughout our day and night. It allows us to work, play and rest. Changing vibrational frequencies are what we all experience each moment. Things or environments that vibrate at a lower level have less energy (or Qi) and sometimes can even drain a person's energy. Things that vibrate at a higher vibrational level increase your life force energy and makes you feel GOOD.

When you have treatment with Master Hai, he will scan your body for blocks and begin discovering what is not flowing properly. His sensitive abilities allow him to see where there may be dark areas, or blocks, in your system and where the Qi is not flowing optimally. He gently will begin to awaken the dormant areas with life energy by touching pressure points on your body. He will ask you to turn over a few times during treatment so that he can check all areas and treat each side accordingly.

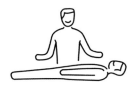

When Master Hai is treating you, it is best not to talk, but to just relax so he can do his job best. He often will pinch the tips of your toes and fingertips to push the Qi into your body through your body's meridians (pathways of energy).

Depending on how blocked the meridian pathway may be, will then determine how much Qi he will transmit into you. You may feel a heat sensation and most say it is warm and comforting. In the first few sessions he will check all areas of your system to determine what is best for you. If you feel pain or discomfort you can let him know, however, he probably will already sense what is hurting you before you tell him.

Most find that wearing comfortable clothing like sweat pants, or unrestrictive garments seems to be ideal. Being prepared with comfortable underwear garments under your clothes is always a good idea if he needs to see your whole body. Wearing tight jeans or pants would not be wise as they restrict flow.

A series of treatments is always beneficial as the body's memory can often be stubborn. Each jolt of healing Qi from Master Hai tends to back off the negative energy in your body and send it back where it came from. Every human body is different and everyone will experience different results based on their condition and dedication to their health. Taking the responsibility for your health is the first step to wellness and often that can include lifestyle changes in addition to treatments. Most of his patients see him regularly for protection and prevention, as his schedule permits. Newer patients have such amazing results that they request more appointments for additional support and continuation of the progress.

After treatment, it is often recommended to rest, drink plenty of fresh clean water to flush the system, and to meditate to preserve the person's energy.

Treatments vary in length of time depending on the patient's needs. On the average, he spends about 20-30 minutes with each patient depending on the type of block and severity of the issues.

Patients are encouraged to wait in the office after treatment to allow the Qi (high-voltage healing energy) that he has transmitted into their body to absorb and take effect. This is called "sitting".

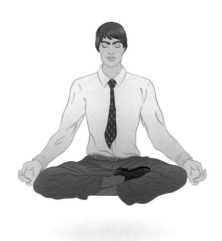

Sitting is best described as a deeper meditative state, in which a patient does not interact with the other people in the room. A person shuts his eyes, puts the focus within his being, and protects his newly gifted energy and field of light (aura). The waiting room in Master Hai's office is like a peaceful sanctuary with many people sitting with their eyes closed and peaceful! The experience is phenomenal because it is a safe haven in a busy world of diverse changes and negative energies. When you are in his office, all you feel is clarity and peace.

Exchanging energy with other people is something we all do on a daily basis to get our needs met, to communicate ideas, or learn new concepts. Learning to be still and quiet within takes practice and effort.

We are always going "out there" for something, aren't we? The search for "something" out there can be endless, exhaustive, and illusionary. We look for love "out there" or outside ourselves, when it is within us right NOW. We mindlessly surf the Internet or watch movie after movie for distraction when all we were searching for is INSIDE.

When we come home to our inner self and take time to listen to our soul, it is a priceless blessing.

Meditation teaches a person to cultivate and conserve the precious commodity of our life, our personal energy. We pull our energy IN, versus always putting it OUT. Meditative states, or sitting, are an encouraged practice that helps a person to be in charge of how they direct their valuable energy. Cultivating a quiet peace within that always exists is what our soul is searching for daily. We often plug into this, or that, and both spectrums are often only temporary fixes or experiences that leave us unbalanced. Find your center within and visit your vast inner world where there is a cherished vault of wisdom and answers waiting for you. Stillness and quiet become the mindless vacation you always wanted to take and can afford!

The body is a complex mechanism and we are always seeking to learn how to best care for it. What works for one person, may not be good for another. Some people may have unusual food allergies while others may be lactose intolerant. Learning what is best for YOU is the great fresh start to feeling better and looking your best. Making an investment in your health is often something that we forget to do because we are always busy or taking care of other's needs. When you make the commitment to dedicate yourself to improving your life and seek out what is best for you, then miraculously new doors of opportunities will swing open to support you.

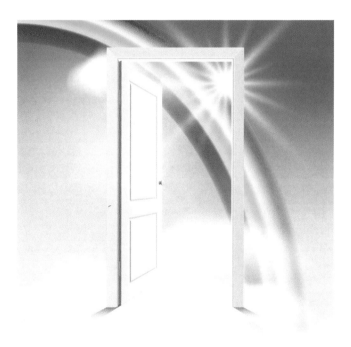

Often people ask, "Do the treatments hurt?" Sometimes, yes, you are going to feel slightly uncomfortable as your body reacts to his energy force. However, the results far outweigh the temporary discomfort.

Many people travel to their appointment alone or on their own. I would recommend to have someone else drive you if you can, however, it is not necessary. I suggest that because after you have a treatment you will want to save the energy you just received for yourself and not rush hour's crazy driving conditions! I would ask a good friend or family member to drive you to and from the appointment, especially if you are not feeling well or have a severe issue. Always think safety first and make good decisions.

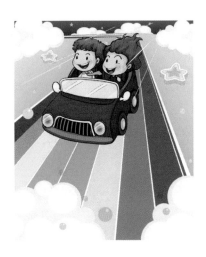

My personal treatments over the past decades with Master Hai have varied from extreme bliss and feeling like I am in heaven to a combination of slightly torturous moments where my brain's pain signals were firing off as nerves were reignited. Everyone is different and no patient is going to have the same experience in the treatment or results. There are no guarantees in this lifetime of anything, as you know, however, the general consensus from his patients is that whatever measures were necessary to correct the imbalances were well worth it. The overall feeling of wellness and rejuvenation begins after the first treatment for most patients. Some patients feel worse after treatments because all the toxins are leaving their bodies and this cleansing process can be uncomfortable.

For example, I have had treatments that were along the lines of deeper emotional cleansing of past baggage and trauma. I used to carry all the painful emotional traumas in my body's storage centers throughout my system. They were heavy, dark memories of emotional pain that lay dormant and hidden in my body.

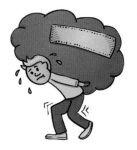

I would bring the heavy bags of emotional wounds with me into every new life moment and relationship because I had never fully dealt with them.

In 2017, I dedicated my time and energy to healing my inner self and this included healing the deeper emotional wounds I didn't want to feel or process.

Previous treatments with Master Hai were more focused on primarily physical symptoms I suffered from. I had never really focused or asked for help with my emotional, mental and inner world. However, I made the commitment to cleanse my inner world from negative vibrations that I carried with me. I realized I had to heal myself and take the heavy emotional pains out of my soul's memory because it was affecting all areas of my life.

As I began the healing processes with Master Hai, the treatments magnified the old past wounds, forcing me to feel them and then get rid of them so they would be gone forever. I would sob so deeply in my soul that I thought my head was going to pop off!

I hid the emotional wounds so deeply in my being because I had learned to cope that way as a defensive default mechanism. I think we all do that to a certain extent because we feel we have to march on and keep going on in life. Grieving and loss are very difficult for us humans to process and yet it is what we all go through cyclically as we move through this planetary existence from the day we are born.

I had to process the old, past emotional wounds very slowly, one layer at a time or I would have been overloaded. I had layers upon layers of emotional memories that I could not either deal with that had to be faced and felt. I had memories with each wave of emotion that made me feel like I was not in the moment, but reliving the past that I never allowed myself to feel or be present in. The blocked or stuck emotional memories in my body were affecting all areas of my life and once they were processed, they were finally gone. I felt free.

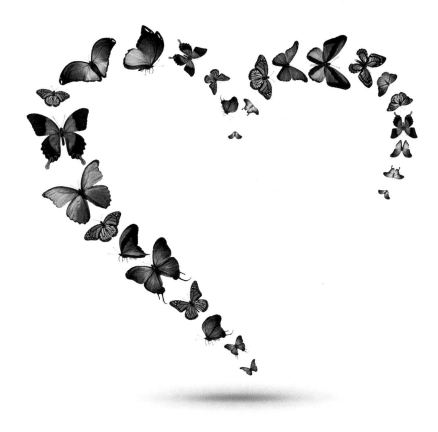

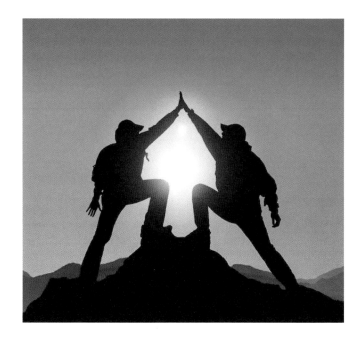

My experiences and moments with Master Hai have been the greatest gifts I have been blessed with in my lifetime. He is constantly and consistently showing me a new awareness of his abilities as I witness the miracles he performs in his office setting on a daily basis. My mind has been blown many times with a new awareness of his abilities that I never knew existed until that very moment. Master Hai has blessed my family and me in so many ways that I am in awe of his constant flow of love and strength. He has been there for me in the darkest times on my journey and taken my hand to help me get through to reach the light again.

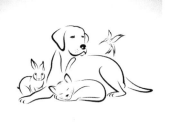 Master Hai even heals pets and animals! Precious animals that cannot talk to tell us they are suffering sometimes need a Qi tune-up as well. I began to realize that all living things could benefit from removing stagnant, blocking Qi energy from their system.

An example of removing old, stagnant negative Qi is to consider the busy gardener who pulls the weeds and undesirables from the freshly growing vegetable garden so that new life can begin again. Another analogy to help you understand the concept is when you last cleaned your closet or garage and tossed away anything that wasn't being used regularly and noticed the clear and open area's energy.

Imagine, if you will, the concept of depression and anxiety and how our society will hand you a cocktail of pills to remedy any type of fatigue symptoms. Now imagine if what you were suffering from was only adrenaline gland burn-out from recent stresses you experienced and that you don't need a pill that may clog your liver. What if the chain reaction of taking the pill caused your body more problems and now you need surgery because your organs are failing? Then, you hear of a miracle worker named Master Hai who can revitalize your organs. Then, you get healed by him and have so much energy you are taking martial arts classes 3X a week!

This is a true story of just one of his patients who received the miracle healing from Master Hai. I want to share more with you in later chapters. My point in mentioning this story is to express the concept that often what our symptoms are can be camouflaged or masked by other reasons that perhaps don't even relate with any diagnosis. How would we truly know? Master Hai has a gift that allows him to see beyond the symptoms to the core of the problem.

For example, many people suffer from stress-related conditions where too much cortisone is being released into the body when the body's emergency signals are being overly utilized from the stress. This toxic process begins to break down the body's system like a demon trying to steal your soul. Some reach for the bottle, drugs, or worse, they long for death. Longing just for a temporarily release from the constant tormenting pain that plagues them relentlessly. The vicious cycle begins with the person trying to cope with their issues with harsh pharmaceuticals, or numbing narcotics, to get temporary relief, which can often cause further difficulties.

Like I said before, pain in the body is for a reason. It is a signal to your brain that something is not quite right. Masking the pain is disastrous because now you are numb to the signals and the problem within is bubbling within like a volcano ready to erupt.

As a person gets weaker and feels more fatigue, then their aura gets weaker. The aura is the magnetic field that surrounds you that keeps the bad guys out and negative energies at bay. Some of Master Hai's patients call it an "attack" when their aura has lowered and they are more susceptible to the negative energies of the planet. A full-blown attack can make you feel like you are fighting for your life as lower entities can enter and wreck havoc on your being.

This is a spiritual world and the darker side loves chaos, pain and torturing victims. Master Hai fights the dark side every day and wins. He says we have to fight till the end and each day is different.

Praying, meditating, and taking care of the body creates the healing environment for the souls that came to this planet to learn and love. Highly sensitive people, like myself, are more susceptible to all the vibrations on the planet and tend to absorb the suffering of others if they are exposed to them for any amount of time. It can almost feel like you can feel their pain too, and the other person isn't even aware of the depth of your suffering you experience being connected to them or near them.

Each day as I enter Master Hai's office I pray first and ask God to fill me with the Holy Spirit and to use me as an instrument of His Love. I ask God to talk for me, tell me what to do, and where to be at any moment for proper flow. I ask God for an open mind of gratitude and humility so that I leave his office each day knowing I did my best. After leaving his office I thank God for all I was gifted to witness and for having the privilege and opportunity to be there.

I want to share with you now in great detail as much as I can to give you insight into Master Hai's world, the miracle healer that I met in California.

"I cannot wake you up,
or make you wake up.

You must choose to wake up…
yourself."

Master Hai

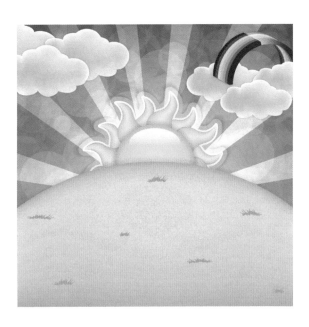

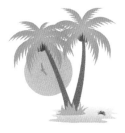

Newport Beach, California

In January of 2017, I travelled from Denver, Colorado to Newport Beach, California to see Master Hai for treatments. I never went back to Colorado. Master Hai offered me a place in his world and I accepted. It was the best decision I ever made to stay in California with Master Hai, and also the greatest sacrifice because I had to leave my family and loved ones.

Master Hai was seeing patients in a semi-retired setting when I returned. I initially just came to California to have my usual "check-up and tune-up" treatments, however, when I realized the atmosphere he was offering was more open than it ever was before to me, I did not want to leave him. I felt divinely led to his office and to him. My inner soul was telling me that I was going to have a greater learning experience with Master Hai this time. It would be the experience of my life and fulfill my destiny.

Willie Wonka and the Chocolate Factory is one of my absolute favorite movies of all time. In the movie, a character named Charlie wins the "Golden Ticket" and the opportunity to see how Mr. Wonka makes his special chocolate. Only a few chosen ones are invited into his sacred laboratory. When Master Hai said I could come observe him perform miracles, I was overjoyed with delight and happiness. It felt like I had won the Golden ticket!

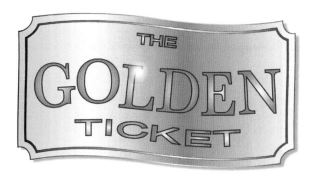

I recalled many years ago when Master Hai had to leave the country and all his patients missed him so much as they scrambled to try and find someone who did what he does and could not. It was a great test. I have found and met various QiGong Masters who could offer some levels of relief, however, they did not have the high-voltage Qi energy that Master Hai is blessed with. Every healer has different gifts and methods, just as every NBA player has different talents and moves. All are not made the same. It was during that search to try and replace him that I deeply realized and discovered how powerful Master Hai is because I could not find a healer who even came close to his level of Power.

I would place him on a cosmic level of having Supernatural Powers that also includes clairvoyance and ability to see the third dimension of the Spirit World.

I promised myself that if Master Hai ever returned back to this country, I would do everything I could to see him more often and learn from him. Well, thankfully he did return. I still vividly remember the phone call many years ago when he phoned me personally and said I could come see him. I was living in Hawaii at the time and was suffering from a debilitating case of sciatica that made it difficult to walk, brush my teeth, bathe, sit, or sleep. The discs in my back were initially injured in a car accident decades ago and the fall-out issues were discouraging as I tried to recover on all levels. The symptoms would reoccur during stressful life phases or also being around other people's lower energy because of my sensitivities.

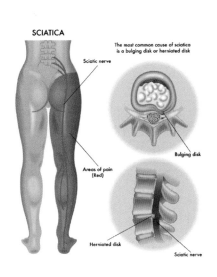

Sciatica is a fairly common type of pain affecting the largest nerve in the body called the sciatic nerve. The nerve goes from the lower back down each leg. It is caused by usually a disc herniation directly pressing on the nerve. I have had to deal with the debilitating sharp pains ever since I had a car accident many years ago. When I am under great stress or emotional pain, the sciatica would make it difficult for me to do the most simple of tasks.

Periodic treatments after the major car accident were life-saving sessions with Master Hai that alleviated the pain and issues so my injured body could heal. I needed the occasional follow-up treatments to keep the issues at bay and they were effective as my entire being was slowly transformed over the years.

I was deeply suffering and in daily pain before I met Master Hai. Western medicine did not have any solutions that worked for me. I tried everything. I spent many years with limiting solutions of orthopedic surgeons, specialists, physical therapists, and holistic healers. I spent a lot of money and time and felt like I was just documenting my issues. They would ask a bunch of questions, diagnose me, and write a prescription for steroids and pills that I never took. I knew any pill would make my situation worse and just clog my liver as temporary Band-Aid fixes.

Master Hai healed me from that phase of my life when I experienced the worse sciatica pain I had ever had in my life. He took all the pain away in about three treatments over a two-week span of time. Years of suffering and pain were gone in two weeks. I was able to walk again without the shooting pains down my left leg and spine. I could rest better and sit longer. Master Hai performed a miracle on me again and I recall the high-voltage energy shooting through my legs as he worked on me. I think I jumped on the table a few times as the power of the energy current he transmits jolted the negative energy out of me. It felt like a zapping of my synapses that entered my being on a cellular level and when he was finished I felt complete bliss.

I will never forget when I saw him for the first time in so many years (he had been overseas for a long time) because he looked at me in the eyes and said, "I can fix this."

The treatments were intense and such a blessing for me and I was set free from the pain.

My thoughts are that as a person goes through life anything can occur or happen that affects a person's health, stress levels and being. The body's system is a delicate, brilliant machinery that can be affected by the earth's energies and the universe's demands. Knowing such a gifted Master is a blessing that I will never take for granted because I am so appreciative for the assistance he has given me in my life.

Getting to see Master Hai, after not seeing him for so many years, was a very emotional experience for me. For me, when I even get near his energy field, I begin weeping with gratitude and humility. I feel his beautiful soul; his love, his power and just tear with emotion uncontrollably. Often I fall to my knees in great respect for all that he has done for me since I met him.

I could write an entire other book about all the blessings he has gifted me, and I would call it "Billions of Blessings"!

I say it is God working through Master Hai to perform these acts of great healing. In my opinion, I think we can all call on God to help us help each other; we just don't do it enough. Master Hai says he stays in constant contact with God. He says that is where all the Power comes from. He teaches those around him to go directly to Source, or God, for all their answers. Master Hai encourages all to develop and cultivate a relationship with God because that is where all their answers are. Building that dynamic relationship with God and discovering the Power within is our purpose. He says anyone can recover from anything, including addictions, and destitute conditions of suffering…with the Power of God.

Each day I was able to spend with Master Hai drew me closer to all I ever imagined life could be with the witnessing of miracles being performed daily. His abilities were being revealed to me and what this universe was capable of and really about. I believe in the Power of the Mind, the Power of our Source's Love for all of us, and the Power of God within.

Master Hai has been a vast learning experience that could not be taught in an educational formal school setting or by anyone, other than him. My job was to show up and observe as he healed patient after patient with a seemingly endless reservoir of energy that replenished as quickly as he transferred it away. A person cannot put this man in a box and describe him with any limitations of any kind.

Since January of 2017, I have been blessed with experiencing Master Hai in high-definition perform his miracles in his office setting. It is the most awesome experience ever.

I witness the many patients walk into the office with dark eyes and faces that are etched with pain and discomfort. Some have been on the edge of death and they didn't even know it. He deals with many severe cases that either Western medicine could not cure or surgery would leave them worse. When the patient walks in, I can feel the weight of their pain in their body.

After Master Hai treats the patient, then I witness the patient leave the office with a facial expression filled with peace, light, and a sparkly glow. His healing leaves a person with a heavenly glow that only could be described as "Master Hai's Glow". The glow makes you feel like you are in another world, because you are. If that powerful glow feeling could be trademarked, bottled and sold, it would be a multi-billion dollar industry.

I have checked thoroughly, and he has no cords or wires that plug into machines, walls, or that are coming out of his back. He does not plug into anything other than our divine Higher Power. He utilizes only his hands, mind, and the Great Source's Energy that most call God. As I write this I must say that my archaic images and belief systems of what God is, was, or can be, have been elevated to the Billionth Power.

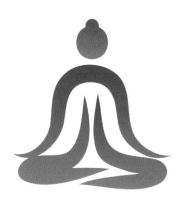

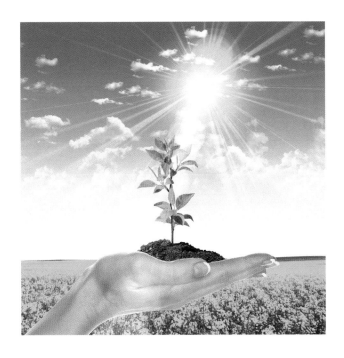

*"What you reap
is what you sow...
this is the main
law of the universe.*

*Focus and direct your precious energy
consciously to produce good results."*

Master Hai

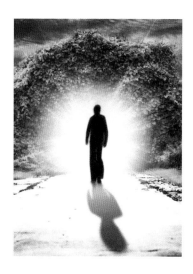

Master Hai

I want to describe Master Hai to you so that you feel like you know him already before you meet him. His nationality is Vietnamese and his full name is Hai Liu, however everyone calls him Master Hai.

I use to catch glimpses of him when I would have the treatments over the decades, as he would be in and out of his medical office rooms, while I sat waiting for my appointment. He always was dressed so professionally with crisp, white shirts and business-like pants.

Now, he dresses adorably casual and comfortable with trendy, fashionable, and colorful threads. He is awesomely modernized for a miracle healer and up-to-date in every way. For example, he favors Nike tennis shoes and adorns many of the colorful styles in his personal shoe collection.

Master Hai is blessed with a beautiful assistant named Malida. She has been loyal and by his side, for decades as well. She is the most precious soul and I am in awe of her as she assists Master Hai each day to treat his patients and perform his miracles. I have learned a great deal from her as she gracefully deals with life's obstacles and challenges with a cheerful finesse. I am forever grateful for her. We all love her immensely.

Master Hai's energy throughout the entire day is consistent. When he leaves the office each day, after treating the many scheduled patients, he doesn't look tired at all. His patients leave the office with a bubbly glow and deep peace. Each day Master Hai calmly exits the office with a big smile and says, "See you tomorrow!"

If you saw him on the street or in a store, you would NEVER know that he is a mystical healer that performs miracles each day for many. He looks so normal, just like a human, like you and me. However, inside that beautiful body and frame is a Power that I have yet found words to describe fully, but I will try for you.

Magnificent, Purity, and the Holy Spirit combined into a force that flows from his being into yours. I witness him working miracles on people each day with great awe.

I want to describe to you what a day in Master Hai's life entails and what it feels like. For example, one day a patient was waiting for treatment in the room next to where I was getting a treatment. Master Hai began treating me when we both heard a deep, loud wailing and screaming that still brings chills to my skin as I write this. He said to me, "Wait here. I will be right back." He exited from the room I was in and shut the door. He then entered the wailing woman's treatment room.

This patient was tortured regularly by this negative entity and it came through her body as her having seizures. They weren't seizures though, they were attacks that were so painful and paralyzing that she often feared losing her life. She credits Master Hai for saving her life and keeping the negative energy away from her body. She suffered most of her life until she met Master Hai and tried everything that the medical world could offer her to no avail. She never knows when she is going to be attacked by the negative energy. The attacks become less and less as she is treated by Master Hai and eventually will be fully controlled.

When Master Hai re-entered the room I was in, he was calm. He put his plastic gloves back on his hands and began to continue treating me, as he said, "That is my day. Sometimes the negative energy is on the whole family and they all have to be treated and protected."

I then had a deeper glimpse of what he was doing, whereas before I saw it as clearly medical. He was a shaman, a holy man, and a protector of souls. He could zap to pieces all types of negative energy with his pure white force of God.

"You are very good at what you do. Does the negative energy try to get the souls until eternity?" I asked. I was visualizing the mystic healer in the movie *The Green Mile* who was so sweet and good that could help the humans with his magical powers, but was often misunderstood and unexplainable.

"Yes, until the end." He said with great seriousness.

I knew he was going to say that. I had to admit I was disappointed because I wanted all the bad in the world to go away right now.

"Even for me, I have to fight the negative energy too. It wants us all," he said this in such a truthful and sweet way that all I could do was take a deep breath and hold back the tears.

I lightened the intense moment by asking him what he keeps in his thermos as he continued the treatment on me with great care and precision. I always wanted to know, "what's in that thermos?" Is it a powerful elixir that if a person drank it would give them the powers he has?! I mean, if he's drinking it, sign me UP!

"Ginger, soy milk, and honey," he replied.
"Ginger tea?" I asked.
"No, just ginger root boiled with water and soy milk and sweetened with raw honey."

You know what's in my fridge now. And lots of it. I add the occasional green tea bag or herbal tea variety, just to spice it up. I bought a little thermos like his that I carry throughout the day and I love it!

I love talking to Master Hai, I love being in his presence, and I love him for helping so many people who suffer greatly. The best part of this experience has been having more time to ask him as many questions as I want. I ask questions until my mind goes blank! I ponder deeply on each of his answers as they always touch my heart and assist my soul's learning. I keep journals of all my experiences with Master Hai. I am always writing as I ponder the Universe's mysteries. I am still discovering my own belief systems; so learning about Master Hai's beliefs allows me to incorporate new ways of thinking.

I think it is important for a person to discover what his or her own beliefs are and the search itself is part of our own personal journey. My dream is to travel the world someday and see all the great mystical areas of the world. My mother did this and her brave spirit encouraged me to have an open mind about God and other cultures. Neither my mother, nor my father, imposed any particular belief system on my psyche. They encouraged me to learn and be open-minded about other's belief systems. They encouraged me to choose my own beliefs that resonated with my heart.

God blessed me this year immensely by gifting me more of Master Hai's time. I feel like the blessed chosen one.

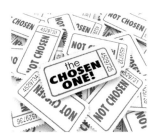

In the past when I would have treatments, I usually just held on tight, like riding a roller coaster, until I am told, "Ok, you can go Pamela, see you next time!"

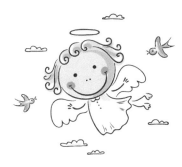

Then, I would leave his office feeling like I was flying, or on Cloud 9, and just incredibly grateful he existed on this planet and that I knew him!

I never had a chance to really experience him, know him, or spend time with him like I do now. Master Hai sometimes sits with us and lets us ask him questions or talk. These are my absolutely favorite moments because I can ask him about foods to eat, spiritual warfare, what the afterlife is like, or anything that I was curious about. His belief systems are that we are experiencing karmic lessons that we must master before we move to the next level or progress. If you feel stuck, it is for a reason, because maybe you are. He shows people the way to set yourself free, claim your life's mission, and start fresh each day. He explains the difference between the inner world and the outer world. Happiness is always available on the inside when you decide to accept it as yours.

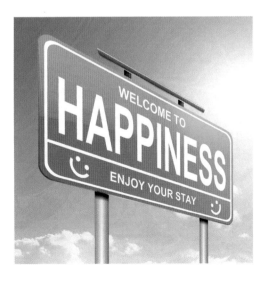

The inner world we have complete control over and we can practice to master it. The outer world we do not have any control over and can let it go. Master Hai says to focus on your own evolution and work on yourself, and let the outer world circle around you without your efforts. He says that focusing within to heal yourself, conserve energy and seek your answers are the ways to happiness.

To be blessed with being able to see him so often this year has been a dream come true.

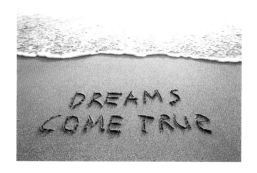

I am learning from a real-life Miracle worker and healer. His sense of humor is priceless and is like music to my ears as his deep laughter radiates in the office throughout the day as he heals each patient. His intelligence level is a combination of brilliance sprinkled with a large dose of down-to-earth common sense.

Even though he is constantly dealing with a major crisis, or emergency, that is seemingly an endless stream of consciousness, he handles them like he is playing tennis, or golf, while he sunbathes his spirit in positivity. He blesses his patients with an added support system that I have never experienced in my life that allows the patient to contact him if they need additional energy, or Qi, after they leave the office.

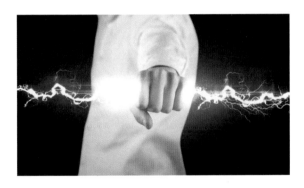

Master Hai has saved my life, and many others lives, in milliseconds with his God-given high-voltage Qi powers that he can transmit via the air without cords or wires!

I know at first it may seem unbelievable what I am sharing with you, and trust me I was the same as you when I was first told about him decades ago. My best friend Brian, who I met in Los Angeles decades ago, told me about Master Hai many years before I finally chose to walk through his door. When Brian would describe what Master Hai did that included the concepts of energy healing work, I figured that Brian had a really good imagination. I thought he was weaving tales of eccentricity that were so far "out there" that didn't jive with my Western medicine upbringing. How could a man heal with his energy, mind, and hands? Wasn't that what Jesus did? Walking on water and parting the Red Seas stories were not in my realm of thinking at that time as I was new to Los Angeles and everybody and everything was quite intimidating, much less someone telling me of their Master who healed people. I think when a person is told about such a human being existing that is healing people with their energy force; it can be hard to believe at first. I had to be completely humbled before I asked Brian, "What was Master Hai's number again?"

When I ended up walking through Master Hai's door many years ago, I was completely shattered in all areas of my life, including, but not limited to: spiritually, mentally, socially, emotionally, financially, and physically. I had been hit by a speeding car going 55mph and t-boned on the driver's side of my car. It was a freak accident. I had just moved to the city of Malibu and was naive to the dangerous curves of Pacific Coast Highway.

I had been through every door that Western medicine offered me that included therapists, surgeons, acupuncturists, specialists, psychiatrists, and physicians. I suffered daily and had somewhat lost hope in this world with very little fight left in me. I felt defeated, lost, and injured.

When I met Master Hai for the first time, I cried deeply. My soul sensed him and his greatness. I recalled he lightly touched my injured body and gently touched my soul in a way that I have never felt before. I felt a great love surge through my entire being and I knew I was going to be ok. I felt in my soul that I had found *him* and I didn't even know who he was. It was an instant deep awareness that every trauma, challenge, or crisis in my entire life had a reason, or purpose, and it was to lead me to meeting Master Hai.

I had many gifts that I needed help understanding and learning how to use, that included clairvoyance, visions, and ability to see the other side. Yes, I felt the third dimension every since I was a young child and a ghost tortured me nightly in my bedroom. Master Hai immediately began healing my mind, body, and soul. He has been a guide and mentor for me as I walk through life's paths of uncertainty. Throughout the decades he has assisted me in many different types of situations, which range from common ailments to real-life emergency situations. Who wouldn't want to go through life with a magical miracle healer that is gifted with powers to help others?

I am blessed to the Billionth Power and I want you to know him too.

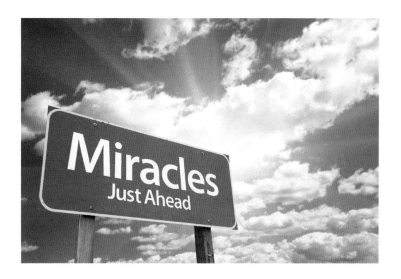

*"Your mind is a garden,
your thoughts are the seeds,
you can grow flowers
or you can grow weeds."*

William Wordsworth

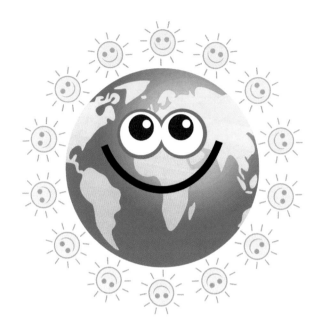

Patient's Stories

All of the patients have a unique and miraculous experience that includes what it took to get them to Master Hai's doorstep, how he has healed them, and what they are like now. The patients are being kept anonymous to protect their privacy and the names have been changed or not utilized at all.

Darth Vader, GO AWAY!!

"He makes Darth Vader in my head go away!" said the ten-year-old waiting in Master Hai's office for his treatment.

My heart dropped as the young boy shared this with me about his personal inner-world because of the way he said it and I wasn't quite sure what he meant. He eagerly opened up to me as we sat on the large couch in the garden. A section of Master Hai's office has a garden where patients can sit before and after treatments to rest.

"Before I met Master Hai, I couldn't do this." He said as he spun his Spiderman keychain around in a circle with his wrist twisting with great energy.

"I couldn't spin anything with my wrist. I had no energy. Now look at what I can do." He continued to spin the keychain excitedly as he continued to share with me.

"Darth Vader in your head?! Does that mean depression? Did you have a Western physician diagnose you before you came here to see Master Hai?" I asked politely and carefully because I was not sure if he would have an answer to my question, but he did and more.

"It is like a darkness that takes over this part of my brain," he said, as he held his hand up to the right side of his head where Darth Vader used to linger uninvited.

"Sure, it doesn't matter what you call it, because Master Hai makes it go away! He made Darth Vader leave in three treatments! He healed my Mom in five treatments. I don't have any more dark thoughts, I sleep better with no nightmares, and I feel more positive and hopeful. My Mom used to be yellow," he said as he spun his key chain vigorously with energy.

"Yellow? You mean jaundice? Liver failure?" I gasped with more wonder and amazement.

"Yes, jaundice and cancer. Now it's gone and her face is bright pink and she looks younger too. Master Hai is amazing, you can go to other doctors if you want, but you will just run back here again because he is the real deal," he said with great feeling and emotion for saving his mother's life.

"How long did it take to heal your Mom?" I asked.

"Less than a year, now she is like brand new and doesn't have anymore fatigue or pain. It's a true miracle."

"Do you tell anyone about Master Hai?"
"Well, I am only ten years old. I don't have any friends really," he paused and looked deeply into my eyes, "and if I did have friends, maybe I would tell them, maybe I wouldn't. How do I know that they would respect his powers and not try and take advantage of him? A guy like this you want to protect. I mean, he saved my Mother's life."

Suddenly this young boy didn't seem ten years old to me at all, he seemed like a very old soul who was wise beyond his earth years.

His mother entered the garden where we sat talking and I asked her about what her son shared with me and she laughed heartily.

"One of the most prestigious cancer institutes in the country diagnosed me with cancer, liver failure, and an early death. I was dying. Then, a friend told me about Master Hai. I came immediately for treatments. A miracle occurred over the series of treatments and I was tested last month and all the cancer is gone. I am going to live. Here, let me show you some before and after photos of my face."

The photos were astonishing, and slightly disturbing, as her face was yellow and wrinkled and the current photo was of her smiling, with a youthful pink glow.

"Master Hai healed you in less than a year?" I asked astonished.

"Yes, I don't have any symptoms at all and I am full of energy now. My father had the cancer and I was told it was hereditary. I was actually with my father at the top cancer institute in the country when he was having treatments and a doctor noticed a lump on my body. The cancer institute did a biopsy immediately and diagnosed me with cancer. It was the death sentence. Now the cancer is gone. When Master Hai first saw me he said he didn't even see the cancer. He said all he envisioned was the body healed," she shared with me as her son playfully rolled on the floor at our feet while spinning his keychain simultaneously and smiling.

I then remembered I had just bought a Star Wars light sword and it was in my car. I bought it to use it as a night light for when I exercised in the evening. I used it to protect me and ward off evening drivers that were not paying attention, as I needed to cross the street. I could easily get another one and I wanted this sweet, young child to have the light sword to ward off Darth Vader forever. He loved it! I was so grateful to meet this precious family. It was amazing to witness and learn about the intense life-changing miracles they experienced from Master Hai.

This sweet child could have lost his mother and the ripple effect of that tragedy could have infiltrated his fate in all his life choices, those he met, and the decisions he would make. The family was beyond grateful and bubbled with joy and happiness. I noticed they had brought a lot of bananas and vegetables in large bags in the office's next room.

"What are the bananas for?" I asked.

"Master Hai charges them with energy for my son's lunches. The vegetables are for us to juice throughout the week and he charges them with his high-voltage Qi energy too. Master Hai recommends fasting a day or so during the week to let the organs rest and cleanse the system. On my fasting days, I juice and drink my nutrients to give my system a rest. I follow all Master Hai's suggestions to assist my body in getting stronger and repairing," she replied.

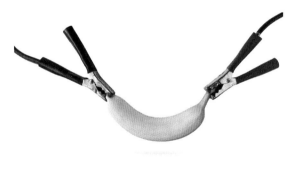

"Super-charged bananas?! Wow! That's awesomely amazing!!" I said with delight.

Master Hai also energetically charges water and necklaces with Qi protection. The concepts we spoke of that day in the office had me contemplating the earth's fragile eco-system and where energy was truly coming from. Did our energy come from our food choices, the sun, or people?

Master Hai says that even food can have bad Qi (energy) if it was manufactured with processed chemicals or colorings. We are eating for energy and some food has no energy to offer you, or it is not digested well in the system. If you are taking good care of your internal digestive system, you don't age as much. It's all on the inside! Eating takes energy and when we eat too much it overworks your system. Extra food that our bodies don't need is stored in your body and affects the ability for your organs to run efficiently. Think less is more and try to limit your meal intake and see how much energy you will have!

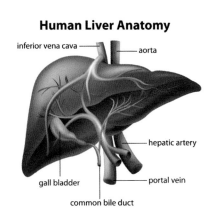

Human Liver Anatomy

inferior vena cava — aorta

hepatic artery

gall bladder — portal vein

common bile duct

The liver is a vital organ located on the right hand side of the belly and is the largest internal organ. It has many functions such as making proteins and blood clotting. It breaks down and detoxifies substances in the body and also acts as a storage unit.

"Why do you care what people think?
Who cares?
Waste no mental energy
on what others may think.
This is your life.
Live it."

Master Hai

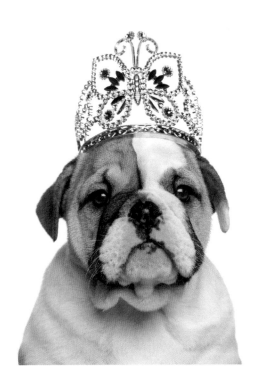

Win-Win...Count me IN!!

Another day I met a gentleman with great presence and full of energy. He was talking to another patient and I overheard what he was saying as I was in a meditative state with my eyes closed.

"Master Hai is amazing. He saved my life. When he left the country for a while, I was in trouble and I am sure all his patients felt the loss when he was gone temporarily. When Master Hai came back, we were talking and catching up. Master Hai told me he heard me call his name from a distance when I was having a torturous attack in the middle of the night. He said he helped me, and well he did, because instantly the pain went away. It was unbelievable that he sensed I needed help from a distance in the middle of the night. He is amazing. He just does what he does and is consistent about protecting those who come to him for assistance. He has saved my life on more than one occasion since I have known him, but that time in the middle of the night was remarkable. It could only be defined as miraculous. I am not kidding, I was in trouble and he was there by just calling his name," the man stated with great gratitude and love.

He exhibited no signs or symptoms of diseases or issues. So I asked him why he was here today.

"Are you kidding me? I would see him everyday if I could! He healed me a long time ago from a back problem and I couldn't walk. Now I golf all the time and have no pain. I see him regularly for preventative reasons and just because I love seeing this guy. He healed me after all the doctors told me I would never walk again. My discs were so compacted I could barely sit and surgery didn't work. After he healed me, I decided that returning to him as often as I could would only be beneficial to my overall health and well-being. Let's face it, from the day we are born, we are challenged with health issues. As we go through life, things happen. The world can be a crazy place so I return for the protection. It's a great investment in oneself. It saves a person money because you have less medical bills. It helps a person make more money because you have more energy. Master Hai makes you so peaceful inside that you are more productive and can make better decisions with your life. It's a win-win. Count me in," he chuckled happily.

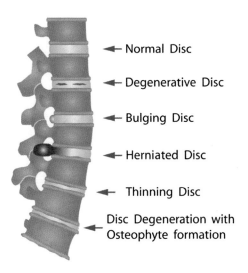

Normal Disc

Degenerative Disc

Bulging Disc

Herniated Disc

Thinning Disc

Disc Degeneration with Osteophyte formation

The spinal cord is a collection of nerves that travels from the bottom of the brain down your back. There are 31 pairs of nerves that leave the spinal cord and go to your arms, legs, chest and abdomen. These nerves allow your brain to give commands to your body's systems.

Moderate exercise and walking are excellent for the spine's health. However, over exercising or rough sports can put too much pressure on the discs and lead to injury. If you can be conscious of how you sit and stand; this is very important for your spine's health. No slouching!

Keep in mind that your bed's mattress and pillows are key elements to protecting your spine and neck. Be sure that they are supportive and have good energy.

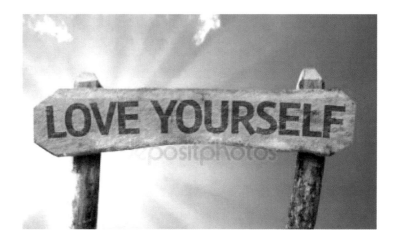

*"Take time
to take care of yourself,
if you don't,
who will?"*

Master Hai

A New Heart

One day a man walked into the office with a shell of a body left and his eyes were darker than I had ever seen in any person on the planet. I think he may have been almost near death, but he was walking into the office with all that he had left.

I sat motionless as I witnessed the miracle healing. The man had multiple blocks in his body that included his heart channel and lungs. His body was shutting down and he made it to the office just in time. Within moments he was in the treatment room with Master Hai and when he came out he was transformed visually and physically. He sat in the chair to let the newly invigorated Qi settle deeply into his system. He looked at me and spoke.

"I almost died today. Master Hai just saved my life. I didn't know what was going on, I just felt strange and I called him and he said to come in right away," he said.

I couldn't believe that he was telling me what he went through today. I would have never known. I saw the transformation, but I had no idea what specifically occurred that day until he spoke. I stared at him with intense curiosity. I was fully aware to keep the speaking to him to a minimum, so that I didn't take any of this man's vital energy. Have you ever been sick or ill and recall how much energy it takes just to talk? It takes energy to speak; we just sometimes take it for granted.

"Your eyes are lit up with a bright light coming out of them and your whole face looks ten years younger now," I stated with awe.

"I feel that way, too. I can't explain how Master Hai performs these miracles. I stopped trying to explain or understand how he does them, a long time ago. All I know is that he just performed a true miracle on me. I told myself that I was going to meet death today and accepted it. I mean to say that dying isn't really dying is it? We just leave our bodies. I will still be here, just in a different form of a spirit. Now I am going to live, it's unbelievable. I could barely drive here when I felt the attack and my body started to shut down. It was my heart. After I called him, I could feel him send energy to help me get here safely. The drive was surreal to me. It was like I was being carried and all the cars moved out of the way for me. I don't remember walking into the office, but here I am now and talking," he said.

"How did he do that?" I asked.

"He recharges the meridians and removes the blocks. Once he puts Qi back in your body and pushes the stagnant negative energy out, it is like a surge of energy. I don't know where he gets the power from, he says God, I just say Thank You Universe and Master Hai! I mean God created him, so his gifts are sacred. He is using them to heal others, not for selfish reasons, because if he wanted to I am sure he could!"

When he said that he made me laugh because it is probably true! Thank God Master Hai is on the Light side of Good! He can see into people's minds, even from a distance. His force can zap a negative entity like Darth Vader to protect a child's mind. Master Hai says that we all have our karmic tests and challenges to overcome what we came here to do. He says that if others are practicing poor behavior or cultivating negativity to just get away from them, not try and control or change them. It saves energy to let them create their own consequences from their actions and just mind your own business and do just your job.

CIRCULATION OF BLOOD THROUGH THE HEART

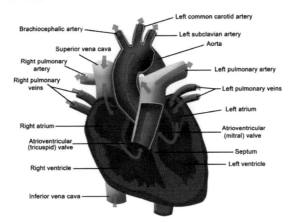

"Blood is everything. Even your skin is blood," says Master Hai.

Blood flows continuously each moment throughout your body. The heart is a muscle that pumps the blood received from the veins into the arteries and delivers oxygen, necessary elements, and nutrients.

Some of the ways to care for your heart is with moderate exercise, meditation, stress-relieving activities, a balanced healthy diet, less salt and regular blood pressure checks.

"You worry too much!
Don't think so much!
Don't be so hard on yourself.
That is a waste of energy.
Just be."

Master Hai

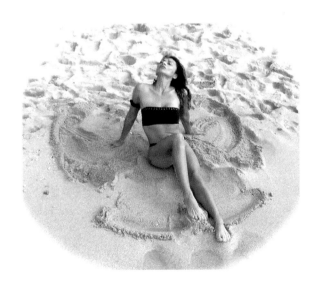

One Kidney, One Life to Live

A gorgeous petite blonde was sitting in the office one day and I had seen her there before, but never had talked to her. Her hair perfectly tossed from left to right when she laughed and spoke so openly about the miracles that Master Hai performed in her life.

I never would have imagined or guessed what this woman had been through. She had one kidney left. Before she met Master Hai, a surgeon removed one of her failing kidneys and she was left close to death. She came to Master Hai with one damaged kidney and very little hope for the future. She described her painful path to me that included physicians, surgeons, and numerous specialists that could not help her.

She has a husband, children and family to live for and found Master Hai just in time. She is now a fully active individual with very few lingering issues. She used to have trouble sleeping, eating, getting out of bed, and had very little energy for the day. After treatments with Master Hai, she now takes various martial arts classes many times a week! She has rebuilt her muscular system with a buff new body. I watched her transformation over the year and it was remarkable. I would see her sometimes in the office and she had a very empty, blank, expressionless face. Some days she seemed to barely be able to hold herself up. As the months of treatments went by, it became hard to recognize her. Her skin tone improved and she was always smiling and laughing with great energy. When she smiles it lights up the room because she is filled with bubbly happiness. She has such a fighting spirit. I knew she was conquering her demons within and winning the battle.

She says that she wouldn't be alive if she hadn't met Master Hai and would do anything he says or suggests to help her continue her upward path of success. She told me that he told her that she didn't need to remove her other kidney because he could have flushed that kidney clean as well. However, she met Master Hai after the one kidney had been removed. He successfully recharges her one kidney that she has left with vital Qi energy regularly to keep her system strong. She returns often to conquer other karmic life issues that she came into the world with that are more complicated inner-world phases. She loves the spirituality that Master Hai offers to his patients.

The kidneys are a pair of bean-shaped organs on either side of your spine. The main function of the kidney is to filter blood, remove wastes, control fluid balance, and maintain electrolyte balances. Kidneys love moderate exercise, a balanced healthy diet, low blood sugar levels, monitoring blood pressure, keeping weight in check, drinking plenty of fresh water, and limiting pharmaceuticals or over-the-counter pills.

ANATOMY OF THE KIDNEY

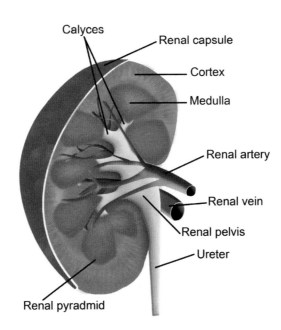

Calyces

Renal capsule

Cortex

Medulla

Renal artery

Renal vein

Renal pelvis

Ureter

Renal pyradmid

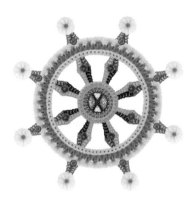

"You can ask my opinion.
You can ask ten other people their opinion.

However,
only you have the karmic responsibility of
the consequences of that decision.

You live with your own consequences and
choices and this creates your karma.

The wheel of karma comes back to you...so
put out the BEST you can!!!"

Master Hai

Whiplash and Whipped cream

A true modern-day Marilyn Monroe with the seductive whisper voice and beautiful facial features describes this amazing patient that I met over a year ago. Often when you come to see Master Hai for treatments you will see many in the waiting room, however, rarely is anyone talking. So you notice people and sometimes you see them again, but you have no idea why they are there or why they are seeing him. That is why I love this job I have right now that allows me to enter into the patient's world and discover new things I never knew existed.

I had seen this woman a few times before and instantly liked her kind eyes, warm smile and sweetness. My spirit was drawn to her instinctively and I was so grateful that I had the opportunity to know her better and consider her to be a great friend. I had never really asked her about her story, and when I finally did, I was surprised that she ever felt sick in her lifetime. She always was so happy and loving when I would experience her. She said her treatments with Master Hai had helped her so much.

"Why did you come here?"

"Whiplash from an accident. I would sit on a recliner all day in great pain. I would eat sweets like whipped cream and cakes and drink lots of caffeinated drinks. You know, for the fake energy and to mask the pain. I felt deep pain in my neck, back, and shoulders. I couldn't do anything. I couldn't get up and I had no motivation or energy," she replied.

"Did you have a Western medical diagnosis? How did you meet Master Hai?" I asked.

"I tried chiropractic treatments, which helped relieve pain temporarily. They mostly offered drugs, which I refused to take. A friend told me about Master Hai and I finally tried him. After just a few treatments, I was better and had more energy. Now I choose to see him as often as I can for the life-supporting energy and the spirituality. I feel like he helps the person overcome the initial issue that brought them to him, then he goes deeper into the karmic and true reasons we came here. I consider Master Hai a teacher and a guide. He encourages me to find my own answers and develop a connection with Source, or God, on my own. He says that the injury was a blessing in disguise that led me to him; otherwise, what would have been my motivator to find him? When you finally meet him, if that is your fate or destiny, you KNOW," she said.

"Know what?" I asked, even though I already knew what she meant. I wanted to hear her words express her truth.

"Know he is going to help you on ALL levels, not just with the physical symptoms that led you to him. With the deeper issues and core problems that perhaps you tried to avoid all your life because they were too complex or overwhelming. Many come from dysfunctional families where the parents either were too stressed to truly love you or care, or were abusive to your soul and you need repairing from within," she smiled and said with great love.

"How do you feel now?" I asked.

"I have so much energy that I take judo classes 3-4 times a week! I also fast a few days a week to give my organs a rest and I don't eat whipped cream and cookies! I have a new outlook on life and I feel like I am exactly where I am supposed to be in life. He even helps me with hot flashes that I experience from time to time, "she said.

"What is that and what does he do?" I asked.

"It feels like a hot flushing that goes through my body and is quite uncomfortable. He gave me special water and when I feel one coming on, I drink it and it goes away in an instant. His energy has the ability to push away any type of negative energy that is trying to attack you or keep you from your soul's higher spiritual path. He protects those that are determined and committed to their highest spiritual path in this lifetime. He uses his God-given gifts to assist those who come to him for help. It is a blessing to have him and every day I thank God for him," as she spoke she cried because of the great love and gratitude she has for him.

"Master Hai has kept me out of pain since I met him and he asks for very little, but a sincere effort for you to do your part. For him to even help me with one day of pain would have been miraculous, but it has now been years and I am speechless. He just keeps giving and helping me and I am forever grateful for what he has done for my family, my fate and me. I love him. He is a true miracle healer, "she said with heartfelt emotion.

"My husband comes to see him as well and thinks the world of him. He has also helped my daughter and my Mother from a distance. I gave him pictures of them and he sends them healing energy and protection to assist them on their journey," she said with gratitude.

Whiplash is a painful neck injury due to a forceful, rapid back-and-forth movement of the neck, like the cracking of a whip. Often when someone is in a car accident this occurs, especially if the impact is a rear-end collision. The neck injury can include headaches, stiffness, vertigo, and dizziness.

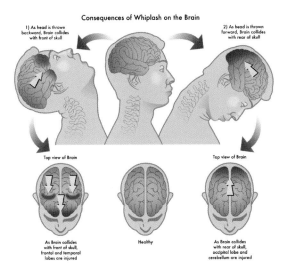

Consequences of Whiplash on the Brain

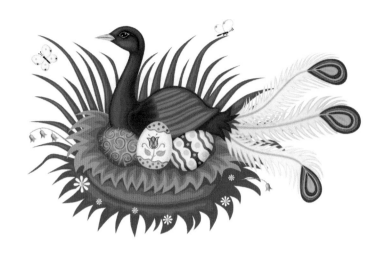

"Just do your job,
let others do their jobs.

Know the difference."

Master Hai

Eating Again!

"Why are you here? You look so healthy and handsome!" I expressed to the beautiful man sitting in the office that I had seen many times before.

"Master Hai helped me so I could eat again. Whenever I used to eat, I would get nausea and vomit or get sick. I lost too much weight and never had any energy to do anything," he said.

"How do you feel now? Can you eat anything or do you have a special diet?" I asked.

"I can eat anything now! I do not have a special diet. I just eat. I used to not be able to digest the food at all and it was very painful after each meal. I have gained weight again and I return to see him whenever I can just for the preventative reasons. I think anyone can benefit from seeing him because his Qi energy is so loving and powerful. I know of others who see him and they don't even have any issues or symptoms, they just enjoy seeing him! He helps in many ways besides ailments that exist, as he can see the entire human being's genetic make-up and soul history," he stated.

"I agree with you completely," I added. "If I could choose to be with only one person on the planet, if I had to, it would be him. He helps a person understand their life path and lessons and learn more loving ways of living. He explains the different levels of the soul's progression so that as a new lesson comes up to learn, he is there to help you master it and move on. He teaches you how to understand your earth family in a loving way so that you can transcend beyond why you chose them and move forward to your true callings. So many of us get stuck in therapy that doesn't work, or repeating old patterns or behaviors that leave us empty because it just rehashes the negative vibrations that were placed on us from unskilled people as we were walking the earth. He removes the old negative vibrations so you can feel your true self and true energy, which can be miraculous. He helps you to feel more calm and peaceful as you go through life. Past family issues or traumas can be overcome with Master Hai's help. He feels that there is no one to blame for the soul's injuries and that it's just the earth's negative forces trying to keep a person down. Everyone on the planet has to contend with the same negative energy on the planet that can come through even those we love especially when they are down or tired. It can feel like you are being attacked and you have to look past the person that the negative energy came through to the source of it and push it back. Master Hai is a light force that pushes away the darkness to protect a person's soul and path."

"I have heard so many amazing stories about what Master Hai has done for so many people and it would blow your mind. He saves lives. He helps the weak and vulnerable. He protects souls. He can transmit assistance from a distance. He saved my friend's life many times and how do you repay that? I mean, we say "thank you", but really, what is the cost of your life? It is immeasurable and he does this all day long for those that come to him for help with sincerity. I am so grateful I met him. I don't even want to think what my life would be like without him," he paused to hold back tears, then smiled.

I didn't have any more questions for him. He said it all that day. And more.

DIGESTIVE SYSTEM

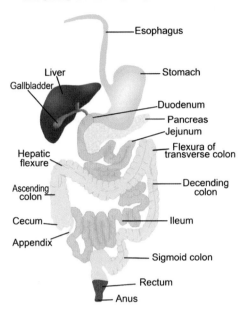

The digestive system is a complex process that turns the food you eat into nutrients that the body can use for energy, cell repair, and growth. It also includes eliminating waste. The three organs that assist the digestive process are the liver, gallbladder, and the pancreas. Chewing your food more actually helps with digestion, so don't gobble it up! Chew slowly and be in the moment fully as you become aware of yourself nourishing your body. Juicing or fasting once a week can be beneficial to allowing your system to rest and cleanse.

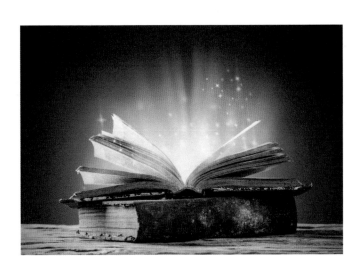

"If you can't sleep at night,
read an inspirational
or spiritual book.

Utilize that valuable time to feed
your soul and mind."

Master Hai

The Acupuncturist's Dilemma

I met more than one practitioner in Master Hai's office who was coming to visit him for aura cleansing because they worked with other peoples' energy all day long.

Call them critters or call them cooties, either way, energy transference for the sensitive practitioner can be problematic. I will try and explain why to the best of my ability. When the practitioner is opening up the other person's meridians or energy pathways, they are creating open portals that can allow for negative energies to get in. If they are open as well when they are opening up the channels, then they are susceptible to the negative energy entering their energy field. It is like taking on someone else's negative energy and it can leave them drained, spun out or worse, vulnerable for an attack.

I have seen more than one physician, acupuncturist, Reiki worker, or energy worker in his office coming to him for cleansing. When they explain why they are there, it always has the same vibration of "OOPS! I did it again! I left myself open and was not paying attention and now I pay the price of pain!" (You can sing that to Brittany Spears song for enlightened effect!)

Remember the last time you went to a place that had lower energy and you left feeling tired, drained, or sad? That was the energy transference effect. Consider the contrasting example of attending a rock concert, or a happy event, and you leave feeling like happy bubbles are coming out of your ears. Now, imagine being a health practitioner and seeing sick patients all day long and you open them up energetically. Where does that energy go? Once the bad energy is off of them, where does it go? Sometimes, the negative energy may have transferred to the health worker or practitioner. We can all be vulnerable to this type of energy transfer, especially if our energy field or aura isn't strong enough. It can create a vortex for the bad energy to travel into your energy field. Many of those that work with other's negative energies all day, periodically come to Master Hai for the clearing of their energy field or cleansing of their aura.

Those that work with other people's negative energy say that the symptoms they experience when they know they are in trouble are the feelings of fatigue, dizziness, or lack of concentration. Some have even considered changing their profession because when they first got into the field they didn't know they were an Empath, or highly sensitive individual. Many have said to me that they chose their particular profession because they love helping people or thought they were choosing the correct path to be of service. However, upon discovering the energy leaks they have of empathy, caring too much, or vulnerability some reconsider their career so they are not opening themselves up on a daily basis to pain.

An emergency room physician at a VA hospital in the area comes to see Master Hai regularly for the clearing off of all the negative vibrations that she is exposed to constantly. However, she initially came to him for organ failure and was dying. She had a ruptured cyst that exploded in her pelvic region and her heart was not strong enough for surgery.

Master Hai was her last hope. He saved her life and that was years ago that he corrected the cyst in her body without surgery. Unbelievable, but true. A true miracle.

As she is telling me her story, and I know that she is a top medical physician, I am completely amazed and in awe. The reality that Master Hai drained her bulging ovarian cyst with a few treatments! She didn't need surgery and now lives to tell about it. Wow! No, Double WOW!!

"Did it hurt to have the treatments?" I asked curiously.

"It felt mildly uncomfortable, however, I figured I was going to die anyway, so I just put it all in God's hands. Miraculously, he healed me a long time ago and now I just return for the beautiful energy he gives me, as well as the spiritual support. I see hardship and pain all day long and I fight the fight with the patients that come into the emergency room to see me. Some days I am so drained and I feel empty. Then, I come to get a treatment with Master Hai and I feel instantly better, rejuvenated and happy. I feel more positive and I sleep and eat better. I love him with all my heart. He saved my life," she said honestly and with great emotion.

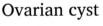

Ovarian cyst

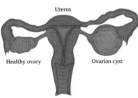

Ovarian cysts are common and are solid or fluid-filled pockets in or on your ovary. They usually are harmless and painless. However, they become a problem when they get too big.

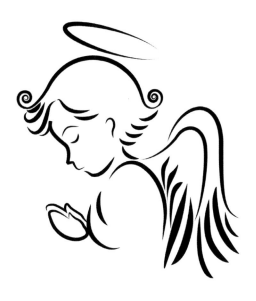

"There is no right way or wrong way to talk to God, or pray. Create a conscious dialogue with God and nurture that relationship first.

All will come naturally after this."

Master Hai

The Angel Appears

When I first met this patient, I knew she was somebody special. I got goose bumps when she smiled at me and I could feel her great spirit. When she appeared in my life it felt like she was an angel watching out for me and all the patients that come in to see Master Hai each day. She is suffering from chronic, painful symptoms and Master Hai assists her in alleviating the pains. Her fight is the true fight because often she is fighting for her life and you wouldn't even know it because she keeps her ailments private and tells very few. I would see her often and she always looked so beautiful and happy. She would talk to me and really listen to me with great care and made me feel so special. I learned so much from her as she guided me through some tough life situations and helped me learn the lessons. She taught me the concept of "putting on my oxygen mask first" in life. She taught me to take care of myself first, or I would not be effective in helping anybody else. She helped me understand the difference between the various vibrational levels that we all live on and everybody has their unique vibration. She encouraged me to protect my vital great energy that Master Hai blessed me with and to channel it and direct it in ways that would benefit myself more. I don't know how she was able to intuit so much in my life situations, but she has great gifts of the spiritual world that allow her to see more than most people can. She expressed often the drain she would feel from the "humans" that always want more everyday and are rarely happy with what they HAVE. She longed for a world that expressed more love and compassion for our fellow humans and prayed earnestly for this vision. Her kindness radiated to all that were blessed with her energy and her wisdom was grand beyond this planetary existence. Her voice is crystal clear and musical to your ears. When you talk to her, you feel like a great soul is listening to you and that she works directly for God. I can feel she is an advanced soul and I can see why the negative forces have tried to get her, because she is helping all who meet her with her energy and light. Her illness is a blessing in disguise because it guided her to help so many by just being present in the room. I am forever grateful for her and I am a stronger because of her great love.

Master Hai is a great protector to the sensitive souls of the planet that unintentionally take on the negativity of others or the planet. I am deeply grateful for Master Hai's gifts that allow the sensitive souls another layer of protection and peace.

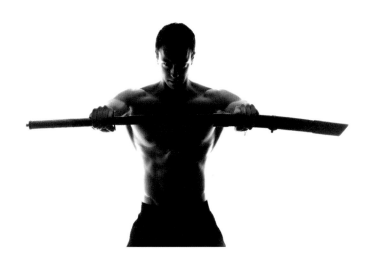

"The negative energy, or thought,
is always out there
trying to attack or bring you down.
Even for me.
Be aware that is the world.

Stay protected
with prayer, good habits, meditation,
and connection to God's power.

Go above the world!"

Master Hai

The Skinny on the Skin

A young female sat peacefully in the office as she shared with me that her entire family had a skin disorder that Master Hai healed. The issue originated in the blood and caused a rash and itchy nightmare that they could find no resolution for in the medical world.

"We tried everything to relieve the painful lesions and rashes that would form on the entire body. My brother had it the worst and now he is completely healed. Master Hai cleansed the blood and all the toxins released in the body naturally and painlessly. We all keep coming back for the spirituality and the great healing powers Master Hai blesses us all with," she said as she sat eating a pear that her father brought for the office staff.

Most patients are so eternally grateful for Master Hai that when they return to see him they bring him gifts. It is a form of gratitude and a kind gesture from the patients' hearts.

I asked her what else she had to deal with and she told me before she met Master Hai that she had no energy and could not do anything. The doctors had labeled it chronic fatigue and gave her pills that did not work at all. They made her more tired and her stomach hurt from them.

"Master Hai told me it was blocks in my system that didn't allow the energy to freely flow. After he released the blocks, I was filled with great energy. I can go to school now, I have more activities in my life and I can exercise. I used to just sleep all day and had very negative thoughts about my future and life. Now I have hope and I love Master Hai so much for giving me this chance at life. He is a true miracle worker," she said.

Her skin was glowing and her energy levels were registering off the charts now! I couldn't imagine this person any other way, but filled with vitality and life!

Master Hai has effectively treated skin cancer in many patients and their families that have come to him with this condition. His energy pushes the toxins out of the body that are trapped in the blood that are causing the problems. When the body naturally flushes itself, then the problem or condition leaves the person's body.

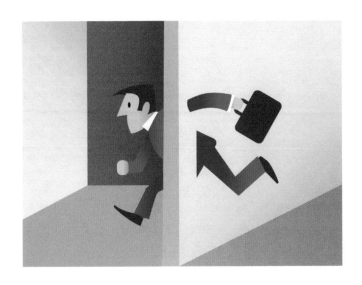

"There is no such thing as reality.
We are all creating it.

Walls are an illusion as well.
We are all connected in spirit."

Master Hai

Flying in from all over the World

How many times have you been asked by a physician, or on a general medical form, about your ancestral history or background? Why do they do this? They are trying to determine if you have any pre-dispositions to any diseases or problems that you may have inherited through your ancestral DNA genetics.

A patient has come to see Master Hai for over 15 years because of her parents and grandparents issues with the heart and having strokes. She never developed any of the issues they did and she made a decision to keep the critters at bay by returning regularly to see him. She flies in from the other side of the country and stays a few weeks to have multiple treatments before she returns back home.

"What are you here for?" I asked.

"Nothing really," she said, "my family has had a lot of problems with their health and by coming to see Master Hai I have not inherited any of their karmic issues or physical problems. I am happy, healthy and productive and I want to stay that way as long as I can. I have told many people about him and I am a firm believer in the power of his miracles. I try to see him a few times a year from across the country. It is worth it to me. It saves me money in the long run by preventing future medical bills or having to take time off work with medical setbacks due my family's long history of illness. I am always healthy and happy," she smiled as she sat in the garden's sunshine.

As she was talking, another patient came to sit by us who flew in from Alaska regularly for a series of treatments for multiple sclerosis (MS). Sometimes she brought her children and family, other times she came alone. She could walk very well, except for a slight limp, which indicated it took her great effort to lift the other leg's muscles to walk.

"Master Hai has given me great relief from this disease and I had tried everything before I met him. He assists me with the travel to come here by sending me protective energy and I find that strangers help me along the way to get here safely. It is a surreal, magical process and I am going to try and come more often to increase the amazing results I am having. There is no cure for this disease. Master Hai increases the blood flow and nerve activity immensely which allow for more Qi or life force energy to surge throughout my body and limbs. I continue to make progress as I dedicate myself to the treatments and do my part with nutrition and rest. I don't think there is anyone out there like him who has the power to do what he does and I am eternally grateful for him," she said.

I met her two kids on one of her trips to Newport Beach this year. She has a young son and daughter that are so precious and adorable. I was able to visit with them and was so impressed with them.

"Do you see Master Hai as well?" I asked the two sweet children.

"No, just our Mom. We just support her and we like to come with her to see Master Hai when we can. It's summer now so school is out and even my Dad came with us this time! Sometimes we stay in a hotel when we come to Newport Beach, however, right now we are in a great condo we found on www.airbnb.com, " he told me.

"Do you watch movies and read while you are here, like a vacation?" I asked.

"Yes! One time I brought a DVD player with me in my backpack and it was so funny. I was crossing the street and it started to play really loudly because I think I accidentally pushed a button on it when I was walking. Everyone started staring at me because my backpack was talking loudly and I couldn't stop to turn it off right then!" he giggled.

"You know California has the best thrift stores and you probably could get a DVD player for less than ten dollars here and then just donate it back when you leave," I suggested. I was picturing this sweet 11-year old boy carrying a DVD player on his back so his family could have entertainment while their loving Mother received treatments. That is true dedication to health. He is willing to carry a heavy metal box through the airport for his beautiful Mama.

"Great idea about the thrift store, I never thought about that! I love Master Hai and all he has done for my Mom. He is the best," he said.

His sister sat with him and they both read the most interesting novels filled with sorcerers and magicians that fight off demons and win. He was showing me his latest book series that he was avidly interested in and I was so impressed with his intellectual abilities. I really enjoyed meeting them after knowing their mother for over a year and only hearing about them.

When I would meet the patient's family after first knowing the patient for some time, it always was emotional for me. I could imagine and feel the stress the family had to go through to get help for their loved one. Master Hai brings in hope, sunshine, new life and ignites the entire family's spirits with happiness.

MULTIPLE SCLEROSIS

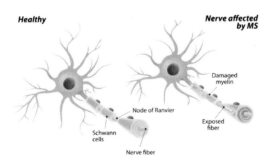

Multiple Sclerosis (MS) is a disease of the central nervous system that disrupts the flow of information within the brain, and between the brain and body. It is considered an autoimmune disease, but the exact cause is not known.

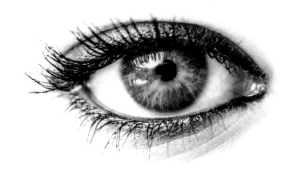

"It only seems BIG
when its in front of your eye
or you are IN the situation.

Step back and look again at your
situation to SEE it more clearly…
then make a new decision."

Master Hai

Achy, Breaky Hands!

Another patient flies in from Alaska regularly and he lives on a boat and is a fisherman by trade. He is the kindest soul you could meet and so gentle in spirit and speech.

"Master Hai heals my hands. I had arthritis so bad that I couldn't even bend my fingers. I couldn't write, hold a book, or get things done very well. I tried everything before I met him and I had just given up and accepted my handicap. A friend of mine told me about him and I flew in immediately to see him. Best decision I ever made in my life. I have no pain anymore and I see him regularly for check-ups and tune-ups. You know, I am in my 70's and the body breaks down, as you get older, however, with Master Hai I have less pain. Sometimes it's instant relief. A person doesn't have to believe or do anything, just show up and let the miracles happen. I live a pretty isolated life on the boat and there are not many doctors around the area when I am on the ocean, so he is a true blessing when I need help. If I text him, he sends me energy and healing through the airwaves. I don't know how he does this, but once he knows you, he can transmit Qi easily when you are in pain or suffering. I don't know what I would do without him. I thank the Great Lord for him everyday. See what I can do now?" he said as he wriggled all his fingers on his hand really quickly without pain.

I could see the knots in his hands where the arthritis had tortured his joints and now they almost seemed to be glowing. He had no more pain and left that day with a huge grateful smile that lit up the whole room.

RHEUMATOID ARTHRITIS

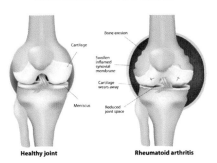

Arthritis has to do with your joints, which is the place where the bones connect. When the cushions on the ends of your bones, called cartilage, wear away it makes the bones rub together. This bone-to-bone friction causes great pain and discomfort.

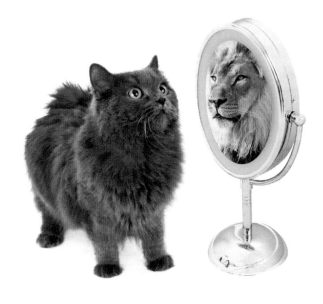

*"The Universe sees everything.
No one gets away with anything.
That is why you let go and let others do
whatever they do…
because it will come back to them!*

*Just focus and work on your
own self-image and give yourself
unconditional love each day."*

Master Hai

Going with the Flow!

A young woman in her early twenties comes to see Master Hai for what she describes as digestive issues. She has suffered with the chronic pain since childhood.

"After I ate, the food would just sit there in my stomach and rot. It wouldn't digest and I could not extract the food's nutrients with my intestines. When I cannot get the nutrients from the food to fuel my body, then I would feel fatigue. I also had blood circulation issues and multiple internal blocks. My hair would fall out because there was no circulation in my scalp. I had blocks all over my intestines that didn't allow for me to go to the bathroom like normal people do. It would be days before the food passed in me, and sometimes not even then. It was extremely painful. I tried everything for relief that included medications, physician's suggestions, and holistic methods and nothing helped. Then, I met Master Hai. He makes everything flow again. My hair is growing back and I feel different. I have more energy and I have hope for my future again," she told me.

As she described her ailments, I sat in disbelief and awe. My thinking was a young girl with a young body, no problems, right? Wrong. A young body can have just as many blocks as an older body may have.

The key is not to wait until the symptoms override your ability to get help in time. The symptoms are what show up to tell you something is not quite right inside your body. It takes time for the symptom to show up and be an indicator of the issue. Usually the issue will get your attention with PAIN!

However, sometimes it is a silent sleeper and creeps up on the person at the last minute when you least expect it. This can be the worst. No early warning signs of the negative energy that has been manifesting in your body unnoticed.

Master Hai can see what you cannot feel and can detect the blocks early, so many patients come to him for preventative reasons only!

"I had relief almost immediately after a few treatments. Now, I just return for the other benefits he offers such as the glow of peace within and the emotional support. I want to come and see him for the rest of my life to help me with whatever I may face in the future. I am not alone anymore, I have a friend, a true miracle healer in my corner," she said.

Circulation

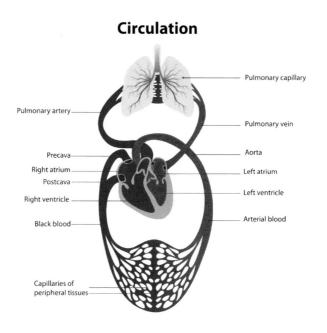

Blood is a liquid fluid that is constantly circulating throughout the body providing nutrients, oxygen, and waste removal. Half of the blood content is composed of red blood cells, white blood cells, and platelets that help with clotting. Blood passes through blood vessels called arteries and veins.

Ancestral Baggage

Another patient had multiple issues as a young girl and then she found Master Hai.

"I wanted to die. I couldn't deal with life. I couldn't focus. I didn't know where to start I felt like I had so many problems. Doctors labeled it depressive disorder, but I knew it was much deeper than that. No pill could cover up or mask what your ancestors left for you to clean up in this lifetime. My family history of manics and imbalances were riddled within my being. I could not separate their stuff from mine. The negative energy attacked me regularly and left me helpless and weak. I know I am an intelligent, beautiful and gifted woman, however I could not tap into my resources because of the issues that drained me on all levels. Master Hai protects me and assists in removing the emotional and spiritual blocks that I have to deal with on a regular basis. I don't know what I would do without him. He offers me relief and a support system that is beyond words or what I could tell you, " she said with great emotion.

I noticed her beauty that radiated the moment she walked into the room that made a person assume she had no problems or issues ever. When she told me of the true issues she faces and battles daily, I could not believe that her inner world was in such torment. It was a true battle for her life with the constant negative attacks on her soul from the other side that her ancestors left for her to deal with. It was almost like she was left with the karmic baggage that they chose not to deal with in their lifetime and it was heavy and painful for her soul.

"I come and sit in the waiting room often just to be near him and feel his energy and to protect me from any attacks. He lets me sit and meditate on the days I need to. It is a pure blessing for me. Otherwise, I would be in room by myself being attacked by spiritual forces. It would look like I was depressed and just laying there. It's not so. I am being attacked and it feels like the spiritual forces are laying on me and sucking the life out of me. Sometimes it's hard to breathe. I use to pray to God for someone to help me when I couldn't get up. God sent me Master Hai who is gifted with a light force that he can send from a distance to save a soul, or in person to expel a negative energy that is manifesting in the body," she said.

As she described her attacks, I could relate as that happened to me often in the past. It felt like a heavy weight was on me and I could not get up. I didn't know how to fight it or what I could do for relief. It is a horrible feeling and it makes you feel inadequate, weak, and lost.

"The negative energy on the planet wants us all. It is always there. Each day we have to spiritually equip ourselves for the fight against the negative thought, negative energy, or negative habit with prayer, God, and the higher forces of light," Master Hai said one day as he was leaving the office.

ANATOMY OF THE BRAIN

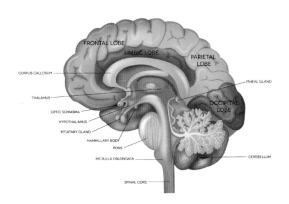

Depression is a mood disorder that has symptoms of feeling sadness or loss of interest. It affects how you feel, think, and behave and can lead to a variety of physical problems.

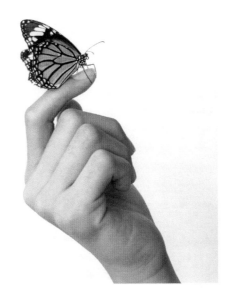

*"Find happiness inside
and it is forever.*

*Find happiness outside
and it is fleeting, changing, and always
moving away."*

Master Hai

Shoulder On!

"I went to a traditional Chinese medicine school to earn my Master's Degree. I always asked the professors and teachers how Master Hai was able to perform his miracles. No one ever could give me an answer. They didn't know either and could not explain it. He just does them. I am so grateful for him."

I met this patient of Master Hai's a few times before, however, had never inquired of what led him to the Miracle Healer.

"I had a bad shoulder. I was about to have surgery and they were going to remove a few ribs to alleviate the pain and imbalances. I never got the surgery. I had heard of Master Hai and finally went to see him. He healed me in one treatment!" he said with a glow in his heart.

I asked him more about his life. He impressed me with his search for answers for himself and the human race, in general. A tall, healthy-looking fellow with deep blue eyes, hungry for knowledge and the thirst for getting it "right" in this lifetime.

"I was fascinated by Master Hai's abilities and it inspired me to work harder in all areas of my life and clean up the messes. I wanted to be free from old baggage, repeating patterns that led nowhere, and discover why I was here. I have seen many so-called healers and energy workers and they are not even close to being in the same league as Master Hai. He is authentic, genuine, and supreme in his powerful ways," he said with intensity.

He explained how his shoulder was a chronic issue and he went to many healers and physicians of Western and Eastern medicine backgrounds.

"I mean, I spent years of my time and money on doctors who could not fix it and healers who tried to help but couldn't. I was in daily pain and it affected all areas of my life. Master Hai pushed the negative energy out that was stuck in my body in one treatment and I have been with him ever since. I come to him for preventative reasons, as well as for the other benefits he offers. When you are in his office, you are lifted into a whole other dimension that is unexplainable with words. He puts you in a meditative state that helps you see the bigger picture and allows you to make better decisions with your life. Life can be a rat race and often draining. His energy lifts you so you can rise above the human condition and you experience who you really are. A pure spirit walking the planet and making decisions on daily basis that affect others lives as well as your own," he said with joy.

I was inspired with this man's insights and explanations because you could tell he really tried hard to work on himself so he could have the best experiences with his life as possible. He didn't take anything for granted and especially was grateful for Master Hai in his life.

Bones of the Shoulder

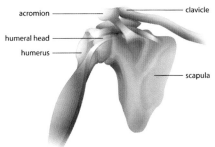

The shoulder is one of the largest joints in the body that is formed where the upper arm bone fits into the scapula, or shoulder blade. It resembles a ball and a pocket that gives range of motion. It is very delicate machinery, be wise and protect your joints and body!

"Just do your best.
Let God do the rest.

Compassion is
for yourself first."

Master Hai

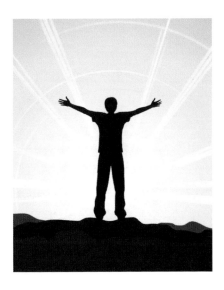

Face and Eyes

"One day I woke up and the entire left side of my face was drooping. I lost the ability to move my facial muscles. It's called Bell's Palsy and it completely stopped my life in its tracks. I could not move forward. It pained me to look in the mirror. It also greatly affected my relationships, how I felt about myself, and how I felt about the world. When a person doesn't feel good, you tend to view the world in a negative way. Your mind projects onto others that they are all having a good time; except you. Sometimes you feel sorry for yourself and get angry quicker for no reason. I went to all the top medical centers and I found no resolution. Then, I met Master Hai. He healed me quickly and my face is normal now. I have no pain and I am happy again. I return to see him every few months, even though I don't have any issues. I return for preventative reasons and for the spiritual lift I receive from the treatments. I have told many of my friends and they come now to see him as well. I travel in from Oregon, so often I come with friends and we share a hotel to save on expenses. It is a time for our health, our future and ourselves when we come to see Master Hai. I would pay him a lot more than he charges because of the benefits he provides and the additional care he gives. His love is endless. He is always giving. He says he doesn't run out of energy. The universe replenishes him immediately and he maintains a balance of constant flowing good energy. He is a conduit of energy and love. I don't know what I would have done without him," said the beautiful woman in the waiting room.

"That's amazing! I also heard that he helped one of your friends with her eyesight and vision," I said.

"Yes, there is no limit as to what Master Hai can do. He is constantly amazing me and helping my friends and family too. We are forever grateful for him," she said with a smile.

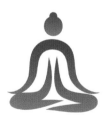

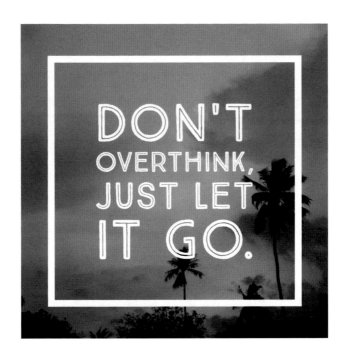

"Keep your mind still and quiet within.
Don't think too much.
Don't think of the past, it's over.
Be in the moment.
That is where all the power is."

Master Hai

Just being Nosy...

An attorney entered the office one day and I had a chance to speak to him about Master Hai. He had the energy of a young boy and moved very swiftly with ease.

"I initially came to see Master Hai for sinus issues that made it hard for me to breathe, especially at night. I am really susceptible to toxins in the air, pollutants, even perfumes. My nose feels like it is blocked and sometimes I would get an infection as well. The painful blocks would make it hard to sleep and then I would suffer from fatigue during the day. It was a chronic condition I suffered with and endured. I tried everything, including over-the-counter medications, as well as specialists. Master Hai regularly treats me for my sensitive nose issues and I have very little problems with them anymore. I have been seeing him for decades and highly recommend him for people who have tried every other remedy under the sun and cannot get relief. He has helped my parents as well," he said with deep conviction.

"Do you see him for any other issues?" I asked.

"Yes, I do. A few years ago I had a low white blood cell count and he fixed that issue before it got out of hand. He is preventative and preservative at the same time! Master Hai encourages me to fast at least once a week to give the organs and digestive system a rest and I have done that for as long as I can remember. One time I was driving a long distance and I was getting really tired. I couldn't stop to rest because I had commitments and so I called him. He sent me powerful Qi energy through the airwaves and I energetically finished the drive. Don't ask me how he does it, he is just blessed with gifts that he uses to help others, not himself. He has spiritual messages that he incorporates into a patient's walk of life that are instrumental to the soul's progression and completion. I don't talk about him much with others because they probably would think I was crazy, but I know what he has done for my family and me. Master Hai is a true blessing," he said with great love.

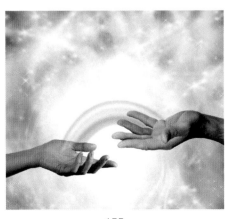

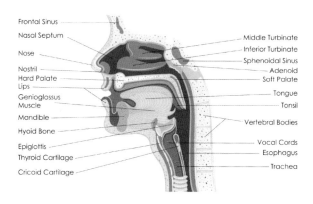

THROAT

The ear, nose, and throat are connected within our skull. The sinuses are four air-filled chambers that empty into the nasal cavity. Sinusitis is an inflammation or swelling of the tissue lining the sinuses.

It can be caused by a common cold, blocked drainage ducts, allergies, and sensitive noses. An irritation to the air cavities within the passages of the nose can cause headaches, fatigue, and great discomfort. The inside of the nose has ridges called turbinates that help humidify and filter the air.

A thin wall called the septum divides the nose into two passageways. These passageways are covered with hairs and mucus that humidify the air. The nose is a gateway for the oxygen that is essential for life.

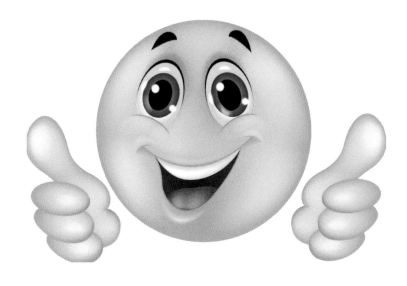

*"Power comes from within.
Practice discipline, focus and a
peaceful mind."*

Master Hai

Epilogue

My journey with Master Hai has been the greatest blessing of my life. I am not sure what I did to deserve such a blessing, but I think it must have been really, really good! I have shared with you only a select few of the many patients' miracle stories. I am very grateful for all the people that blessed me with their valuable time and shared their experiences with me. I feel like my path is complete as I write this paragraph, and that all my dreams have come true. It was a great passion to live this book, and then to have the opportunity to write this book.

I have another dream. That dream is to merge the great scientific standards of Western medicine with the great healing attributes of Eastern medicine. Prior to writing this book, I used to think in terms of Eastern versus Western medicine. I used to compare the two worlds and ask myself which was the better way. After conducting all the research for writing this book, I am now thinking in terms of Eastern AND Western medicine. I have evolved in my thinking and now envision the two worlds merging for the benefit of mankind and for the suffering souls who need alternatives. Both offer insightful solutions and have a great deal to benefit from each other's worlds.

Master Hai is indeed a blessing to many souls. His miracles change a person's fate and the course of their destiny. It takes many lifetimes to enter a realm of miracles, and I have walked through this doorway. I witnessed they do exist.

The human body's system and mind is a complicated and magnificent machinery that we are still discovering new aspects of each day. Chinese medicine sees the body as a whole with connecting organs that all affect each other. Western medicine views the body in a more scientific way. Our body is not just physical though, it is emotional, mental and spiritual. There are many factors that contribute to a person's complete being, that are not entirely scientific.

There are intricate individual patterns that we must master, resolve, and conquer so that we can move onto the next phase of our lives without the heavy baggage in the soul. This lifetime is about your soul. What memories are in your soul, what injuries are in your soul and how to resolve them while you are here so you don't have to carry them into the next lifetime.

Many people are in a hypnotic delusion that they can just physically move to a new place, change their outer world, or buy more stuff to avoid the real reason we came here to earth. They spend lifetimes on empty shopping runs, incomplete relationships or endless Internet channel surfing. When we are able stop, pause and face our selves, it is only then that the true healing can begin.

"Waking Up" or "Awakening" is a brave, courageous action where you consciously choose to confront your reality and begin the cleansing of the soul. It is the greatest gift you can give yourself.

Self-love and self-care are the gifts of waking up. When you realize that this is your one life and no one can do it for you, you must chose to do it for yourself. No one knows the pain you feel inside or outside, just you. When you choose to pause and listen to your body and soul, you awaken.

Master Hai spiritually supports those who choose to awaken and live their life to the fullest.

Every pain you feel, every challenge you have, every thought you think, can be transformed into the most positive experience of your life. It takes courage to ask for help and I congratulate you for all you have done that led you to this moment. We are all in this together and when each of us individually takes responsibility for our soul's authenticity, we positively affect each other consequentially. For those of us who do need assistance in a human form, Master Hai is our life's greatest blessing.

We come in by ourselves, and we leave by ourselves. What you do in between that time is your LIFE. A gift that only YOU can define, with your daily choices and willingness to get it right this time. It is all up to you. It's time now for your miracle to begin...

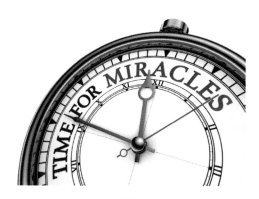

About Pamela

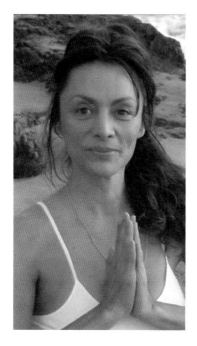

Pamela loves to write spirituality books for all ages. She feels the heart and soul's completion on this earthly plane is our destiny.

Pamela currently attends a University in California and is studying psychology. She plans to earn her doctoral degree within a few years.

Pamela attended a Paralegal college prior to the psychology program, where she earned straight A's in the courses she studied and was offered membership into the Honors Society. Pamela also has earned a Bachelor of Science in Business and Marketing and an Associates Degree in Visual Communications and Design. In addition, she has earned a Personal Training certification and a Nutrition certification from International Sports Sciences Association (ISSA).

Her favorite place is Whole Foods Market® that offers the best and freshest foods, snacks, and juices on the planet.

Pamela's passion is learning about others' experiences in life and how we all overcome our personal challenges and obstacles. Pamela was divinely led to write this book and it was the greatest honor and opportunity ever in her life.

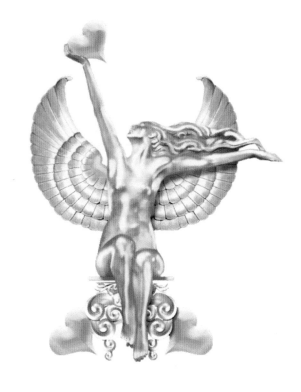

"Ask your Angels to surround you and walk with you all day today."

Pamelarocks

Other books written by Pamelarocks®:

The Rainbow in the Jar
The Pond in the Spiritual Garden
Billions of Illusions
Billions of Illusions: The Sequel

Website: www.Pamelarocks.com

E-mail address:
pamelarockstheworld@gmail.com

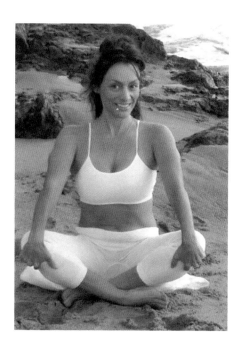

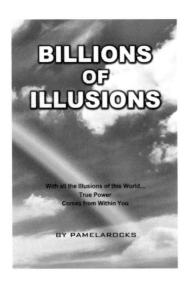

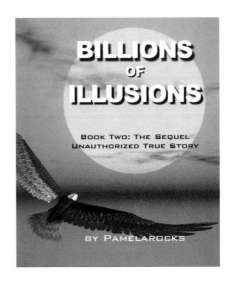

The Pond
in the
Spiritual Garden

Rainbow
in the Jar

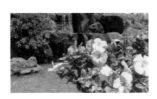

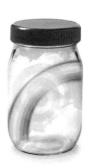

BY PAMELAROCKS

BY PAMELAROCKS

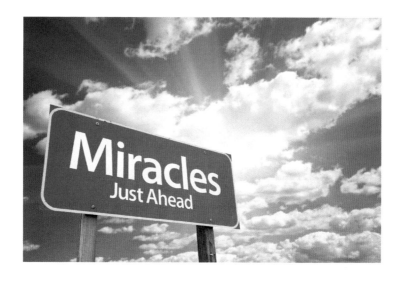

If you or someone you know would like to know more about Master Hai and his miracle treatments, please email directly at:

E-mail address:
<u>miraclehealerincalifornia@gmail.com</u>

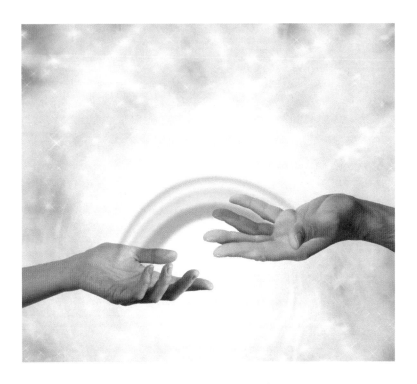

www.miraclehealerincalifornia.com